TRUE OR FALSE?

There is a proven correlation between lack of sleep and weight gain.

True. The latest studies show that sleep loss disrupts a series of complex metabolic and hormonal processes. This can stimulate the production of hormones that regulate appetite, making you feel hungry, even shortly after you've eaten, and causing you to crave fattening foods.

The only way to lose weight is through diet and exercise.

False. A balanced diet and regular exercise are important components of any healthy lifestyle. But they won't eliminate phantom hunger pangs and cravings for rich food. The missing ingredient is sleep.

Staying up late at night burns more calories.

False. Research shows that people who stay up late tend to replace sleep with added calories, often choosing the most fattening foods as their late-night snacks. And even those night owls who do defeat the midnight munchies often wake up the next day with a roaring appetite for more rich and fatty foods.

People who have trouble sleeping are doomed to be overweight.

False. There are many proven methods for getting to sleep more easily and sleeping through the night every night. These, combined with a healthy diet, moderate exercise, and simple relaxation techniques, can help you win your battle with the bulge once and for all.

OTHER BOOKS BY CHERIE CALBOM

The Ultimate Smoothie Book, revised and updated

The Wrinkle Cleanse

The Coconut Diet

The Complete Cancer Cleanse

The Juice Lady's Guide to Juicing for Health

*The Juice Lady's Juicing for High-Level Wellness
and Vibrant Good Looks*

Knock-Out-the-Fat Barbecue and Grilling Cookbook

Juicing for Life

SLEEP AWAY THE POUNDS

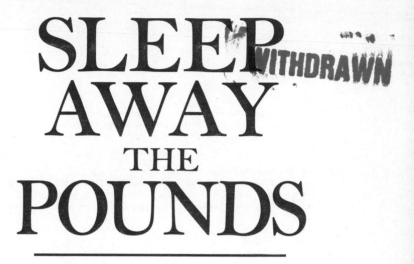

*Optimize Your Sleep
and Reset Your Metabolism
for Maximum Weight Loss*

CHERIE CALBOM, MS,
WITH JOHN CALBOM, MA

Foreword by Stephen Sinatra, MD, author of
The Fast Food Diet and *The Sinatra Solution*

**WELLNESS
CENTRAL**

NEW YORK   BOSTON

Neither this diet program nor any other diet program should be followed without first consulting a health care professional. If you have any special conditions requiring attention, you should consult with your health care professional regularly regarding possible modification of the program contained in this book.

Wellness Central
Hachette Book Group USA
237 Park Avenue
New York, NY 10017

Visit our Web site at www.HachetteBookGroupUSA.com.

Printed in the United States of America

Originally published in hardcover by Hachette Book Group USA

First Trade Edition: October 2007
10 9 8 7 6 5 4 3 2 1

Wellness Central is an imprint of Grand Central Publishing.
The Wellness Central name and logo is a trademark of Hachette Book Group USA, Inc.

The Library of Congress has cataloged the hardcover edition as follows:
    Calbom, Cherie.
Sleep away the pounds : optimize your sleep and reset your metabolism for maximum weight loss / Cherie Calbom, with John Calbom.—1st ed.
        p.   cm.
    Includes index.
    ISBN-13: 978-0-446-57942-1
    ISBN-10: 0-446-57942-4
    1. Weight loss.   2. Sleep—Physiological aspects.   3. Sleep—Health aspects.   I. Calbom, John.
II. Title.
RC547.C33   2007
616.89'498—dc22   2006018551

    ISBN 978-0-446-69766-8 (pbk.)

Book design by Giorgetta Bell McRee

CONTENTS

FOREWORD.. vii

INTRODUCTION xi

CHAPTER ONE: *Sleeping Can Make You Slim* 1

CHAPTER TWO: *Step One: Your Best Sleep Now*................ 27

CHAPTER THREE: *Step Two: Quieting the Mind,
Restoring the Soul* 44

CHAPTER FOUR: *Step Three: Exercising for Better Sleep
and a Slimmer You* 79

CHAPTER FIVE: *Step Four: The Optimum Diet for Sound Sleep
and Super Weight Loss* 99

CHAPTER SIX: *Extra Help for Balancing Your
Body Chemistry* 120

CHAPTER SEVEN: *Solutions for Insomnia and Other Sleep Disorders* 137

CHAPTER EIGHT: *The 21-Day Sleep Away the Pounds Menu Plan* 164

CONCLUSION: *Summing It Up, Sending You Off!* 197

ACKNOWLEDGMENTS 200

RESOURCES 202

REFERENCES 208

INDEX 217

FOREWORD

The idea that one could lose weight while sleeping definitely sounds like a notion that is too far-fetched to believe. Yet the theories put forth in *Sleep Away the Pounds* are so compatible with my research and philosophy on cellular energy, the heart, and your health, that they make perfect sense. In this book Cherie and John Calbom present a comprehensive analysis of the important link between poor sleep and weight gain and outline a clear program that tells readers how to reverse both. Yet this book is not simply a quest to improve one's quality of sleep and drop a few pounds. It's also an analysis of the metabolic, physical, psychological, emotional, and spiritual planes that impact our daily lives.

The epidemic rates of both obesity and sleep problems make them health and lifestyle issues that are of the utmost importance. I've been acutely aware of these problems since my medical school days in the 1970s. As a cardiologist practicing medicine for more than thirty years, it's no surprise that the bulk of my day is about dealing with the consequences of obesity. I must say that I've also seen more than my fair share of sleep-deprived patients. Whether it's a problem of falling asleep or staying asleep, most of us know how sleep disruption can affect our waking hours, but until now, many people have not realized how much it can contribute to weight gain.

The link between sleep and weight loss involves complex metabolic pathways. And the Calboms discuss in straightforward detail the body's varied hormonal interactions and how they affect our rest and recovery—and metabolism. They provide the reader with a simple-to-understand discussion of growth hormone, cortisol (nicknamed the "vigilance hormone"), insulin, leptin, thyroid, and other hormones. There is also content on how various foods we eat can adversely affect the thyroid, a gland that needs to be functioning optimally for quality sleep.

The Calboms point out that blood sugar swings are another common cause of sleeplessness. Many folks don't realize that late-night snacking—particularly on sugary foods—can literally leave us counting sheep all night long, especially if there's any caffeine onboard to overstimulate the brain.

Sugar and caffeine are only a couple of a host of toxic chemical culprits that rob the cells of vital energy, making rest and weight loss virtually impossible. And reducing the amount of these substances in the body is key for success. The Calboms also wisely inform the reader about the need to detoxify the body to achieve optimum health, something I've been writing about for years in my own books, as well as in my monthly newsletter "Health, Healing and Nutrition." Detoxification is essential to a good night's sleep, and the balanced metabolism and weight loss that accompany a healthy body. In *Sleep Away the Pounds* you'll find a discussion on how even minimum liver dysfunction impairs a good night's sleep, as well as how to "detox" your liver and colon for weight loss.

It's my experience when I counsel patients that detoxification is not a subject or recommendation presented by conventionally trained medical doctors. But physicians trained in what we often refer to as complementary or alternative medicine—particularly naturopaths—study and use detoxification interventions as a way of healing the body.

The Calboms, too, recognize the vital importance of detoxification and are quite astute in placing such emphasis on it. Many contaminants can adversely affect mitochondrial function—which most health professionals now recognize is the key to health and longevity. The mitochondria are microscopic organelles in the cells that generate adenosine triphosphate (better known as ATP) for energy production. And because mitochondria are a part of our bodies' DNA that is particularly fragile, when they become vulnerable from things like oxidative stress and environmental toxins, they struggle to produce enough ATP to sustain important cellular processes throughout the body, eventually causing a host of health problems.

Indeed, the Calboms point out that poor cellular health can often lead to problems like sluggish metabolism, poor digestion, hormonal imbalance, and nonrestorative sleep—all of which impede weight loss efforts. Thus, the recommendations for juicing, colon cleansing therapies, high-fiber diets, and healthy food choices outlined in this book are major steps in the detoxification process and play a vital role in reaching one's ideal weight.

It only makes sense that the techniques the authors put forth here to improve sleep quality and quantity will assist the body in restoring itself, and that healthy metabolism and weight will follow if you persist and continue to make healthy lifestyle choices as well. It has been said by many prominent healers that restful sleep is the best antioxidant of all.

Surely, this book is not only for dieters and the sleep-deprived, but is also a useful handbook for the health professional who, like myself, encounters sleep problems and obesity on a daily basis. The Calboms raise intriguing questions and offer sound solutions to benefit anyone who follows the vital program information set forth in *Sleep Away the Pounds*.

—Stephen T. Sinatra, MD, FACC, FACN, CNS, CBT

INTRODUCTION

Are you tired of trying to starve yourself into a smaller size? Are the pounds you've lost for the third or fourth time now starting to creep back on again? Chances are, you're missing a basic fundamental of life. Sleep. It's as important as eating well or exercising, but statistics show that as a society, we are getting less sleep per night than we did a century or even a few decades ago. According to a number of doctors, two chief complaints they hear from their patients are that they don't sleep enough and are gaining weight. And scientists are finding that there is a correlation.

The early bird can't also be the night owl, but that's what many of us are trying to be—both. And instead of getting the worm, we're getting fat. A lack of sleep has been shown to cause weight gain along with a host of other physical problems. And strange as it might sound, there's a growing body of evidence showing that good sleep habits are essential to the success of any weight loss plan.

A succession of recently published studies show that sleep loss disrupts a series of complex and interwoven metabolic and hormonal processes. This can cause a number of the hormones that regulate appetite to get out of whack and trigger a rise in hormones that give you the munchies and cause you to crave fattening foods. This hormonal imbalance makes weight loss far more difficult than it needs to be.

When most people hear the word *hormone,* they think of the sex hormones, such as testosterone or estrogen. Yet these are just two of the many hormones that regulate virtually everything your body does. Hormones have the power to change the messages your brain sends—including some critical ones, such as whether your body should burn fat or keep it around for when food might become scarce, and also which foods you want to eat. Specifically, sleep loss affects levels of hormones that both stimulate and curb the appetite and cause you to crave rich food.

Sleep is the ingredient researchers are pointing to as the missing link in weight loss plans. It could be the reason you've struggled for so long to lose weight and get your appetite under control. When you've completed *Sleep Away the Pounds,* you'll be armed with new information that will enable you to surpass the usual one-, two-, or three-pronged weight loss programs that focus solely on diet, stress reduction, and/or exercise.

In *Sleep Away the Pounds,* you have a revolutionary four-step weight loss plan that's simple to incorporate into your daily life. Equally weighted, the four parts of the plan are a diet that's easy to follow and helps you sleep well, too; stress reduction; exercise; and a fourth key element—a sound sleep regimen.

Many of us have been tempted to think that if we stay up late to work or play, we'll burn up more calories and send the scale moving in the right direction. But research shows that this is simply not true. It's getting more sleep, such as seven to nine hours a night, that's the ticket to a lean body. Researchers have found that people who stay up late tend to replace sleep with added calories and often choose the most fattening foods as their late-night snacks. But even if we eat nothing when we're up late, we're throwing our appetite-regulating hormones out of whack. And that will catch up with us the next day with a roaring appetite for more rich and fattening foods.

If you've struggled to lose weight, or you lose and gain but remain the same size, sleep may be your ticket to the lean body you want. Isn't it time to learn how to get your best sleep starting today? In Step One, you'll discover more than sixty practical tips for a good night's sleep, making this step a super guide for weight loss success.

But that's just the beginning. *Sleep Away the Pounds* is a comprehensive plan that gives you all the steps necessary to lose weight successfully. Step Two includes stress-reduction and relaxation practices that will help you quiet your mind and calm your soul. Stress is a major culprit in weight gain, and stress hormones are responsible for fat deposits, especially around the waistline. Step Three focuses on a variety of practical exercise tips that can help you improve your sleep, burn up calories, and improve muscle tone. Step Four contains dietary advice that includes supplements to help you sleep better and lose weight faster.

With our simple 21-Day Sleep Away the Pounds Menu Plan, you can optimize your sleep and reset your metabolism to achieve maximum weight loss. You should lose about two to three pounds a week. And whether your body has become resistant to hormones that suppress appetite or you have a slow metabolism due to lack of sleep or the wrong dietary choices, the Sleep Away the Pounds Program will help you sensitize your body to appetite-suppressing hormones, balance your blood sugar, and help you become a fat burner again. The same diet that will correct those problems will also help you get a good night's sleep. It's all interrelated, and it's all in the most revolutionary weight loss program now available.

Further, if you're one of the seventy million Americans who haven't been sleeping well, you can experience a better night's sleep. In the pages that follow, you'll discover a host of tips to help you overcome insomnia. We'll discuss the many factors that contribute to poor sleep—including an overactive mind and an imbalanced endocrine system—and help you find solutions to get the restorative sleep your body needs. In Chapter 6, there's help for balancing your adrenal and thyroid glands, and in Chapter 7 you'll find advice for insomnia and sleep disorders, which will help you get to the root of sleepless nights and unrefreshing sleep.

A NEW SLEEP PATTERN FOR A SLIMMER YOU

When you complete this program, you should no longer view sleep as a waste of time. You'll know that sleep is one of your best weight loss buddies. Owning the night will have a completely new meaning: You snooze, you lose! And that's not money, opportunity, or fun. It's weight! But you'll also gain better health, and that will afford you more chances for opportunity, making money, and having fun than you might expect. How simple can that be? As you sleep away on your fluffy pillow, counting little lambs, your body is burning fat and creating hormones that will curb your appetite. And if you've had trouble sleeping, you should be slumbering like a baby before long with our Sleep Away the Pounds Program.

Best of all, you will have changed your biochemistry so that the hormones that make you want to eat a bag of chips before you get out of the grocery store are under control. Your new internal chemistry means a better-functioning metabolism that will burn fat even while you are sleeping. It's effortless. How great is that?

With the groundbreaking steps in *Sleep Away the Pounds* you will improve your hormone balance, fat metabolism, brain function, and health and finally achieve that slimmer physique you've been after. So grab a mug of chamomile tea, curl up with your favorite blanket, and get ready to sleep away all those unwanted pounds—for good!

SLEEP
AWAY
THE
POUNDS

CHAPTER ONE

Sleeping Can Make You Slim

Do you want to be healthy, trim, energetic, and vibrant? You can, with a weight loss secret that's been right under our noses all along. Sleep. That's right. The very thing many of us don't do enough turns out to be key to staying slim.

We may be tempted to think that staying up late will help us burn up more calories and speed our weight loss. But sleep researchers say that this isn't so. Actually, we typically burn a limited number of calories—say, only about fifty in several hours—in the late evening. And we may think that if we cut our sleep short and get up extra early to go to the gym, we'll see the scale move in the right direction. Yet the harder we work out, the more discouraged we can sometimes become, as we remain stuck at a weight plateau. Some of us search for the magic bullet that will help us get rid of those last ten pounds, but it continues to elude us.

Could a good night's sleep be the missing ingredient? Sleep does indeed emerge as an important piece of the weight control puzzle, according to Stanford University sleep researcher Dr. Emmanuel Mignot. He states, "Most people think that sleeping too much contributes to making people fat, but we found the opposite is true."

According to a number of research studies, sleep turns out to be as important to staying in shape as going to the gym, cutting calories, and eating right.

In our frenzy to experience it all, get it all done, manage our universe, and not let a moment escape us, we're missing out on one of life's necessities—a good night's sleep. "We're shifting to a twenty-four-hour-a-day, seven-day-a-week society, and as a result we're increasingly not sleeping like we used to," says Najib T. Ayas of the University of British Columbia. We're really only now starting to understand how that is affecting our weight and our health, and it appears to be a significant factor.

People are the only animals to voluntarily ignore their sleep needs. We've learned to disregard our body's messages when we're tired and needing sleep. We stay up late to work, play, read, socialize, or watch television. Endocrinologist Eve Van Cauter, PhD, who directs the Research Laboratory on Sleep, Chronobiology, and Neuro-endocrinology at the University of Chicago School of Medicine, says, "We're overstepping the boundaries of our biology because we are not wired for sleep deprivation." She adds, "We know the obesity epidemic is due to overeating—too big portions, too much rich food, and too little activity—but why do we crave too much of these rich foods?" Maybe, she says, it's because "we are sleep-deprived and unable to curb our appetites."

Did you know there are hormones that make you hungry and hormones that control your appetite? It's true, and research shows they are significantly influenced by how much sleep you get. Here's what studies have revealed:

- Five major appetite-influencing hormones can get out of whack when you don't get enough sleep, which significantly affects how much food you eat.
- When you are sleep-deprived, your metabolism can really suffer, which causes weight gain.

- Appetite-suppressing hormones and appetite-stimulating hormones are best regulated when you get seven to nine hours of sleep per night.
- You won't tend to crave high-calorie, carbohydrate-rich foods nearly as much when you get adequate, refreshing sleep.
- Sufficient sleep will help you manage your blood sugar more effectively, which helps you manage your appetite. Even one week of sleep deprivation can set off a temporary diabetic effect, causing you to crave sugar and other fattening foods.
- Sleeping in a few extra minutes has its advantages. Research shows that if you increase your sleep by just thirty minutes per night, your chances of losing weight go up exponentially.

If you've thought sleeping was a waste of time, you don't need to feel guilty ever again. When you've finished this chapter, you'll realize it's not only very important to staying in shape, but also crucial to staying healthy. By paying attention to your sleep needs, you can be on your way to losing the weight you want—starting tonight. The entire Sleep Away the Pounds Program is dedicated to helping you get the best sleep possible so you can control the hormones that cause you to want to eat more than you should, curb your cravings for sugar and other fattening foods, balance your blood sugar, jump-start your metabolism, and begin losing weight right away.

THROW OUT YOUR DIET BARS AND GRAB YOUR PILLOW

Have you noticed that when you don't get enough sleep, you want to eat more? Sometimes a whole lot more. It may be time to ask yourself if those nights burning the midnight oil might be altering your metabolism.

Research has shown that sleep-deprived people do indeed eat more food, and they often choose the most fattening fare. "During nights of sleep deprivation, you feel that your eating goes wacky," says Dr. Robert Stickgold, associate professor of psychiatry specializing in sleep research at Harvard. "Up at 2 AM, working on a paper, a steak or pasta is not very attractive. You'll grab the candy bar instead. It probably has to do with the glucose regulation going off. It could be that a good chunk of our epidemic of obesity is actually an epidemic of sleep deprivation."

Is there a correlation between the 65 percent of Americans who are overweight and the 63 percent who, according to the National Sleep Foundation in Washington, DC, say they don't get the recommended eight hours of sleep per night? A growing number of sleep researchers assert that there is.

Since the mid-1960s, the rate of obesity in the United States has nearly tripled, to one in three adults. Over the same period, the US population has deducted, on average, more than an hour from their nightly slumber. We've lost about two hours of sleep since 1910, when the average person slept nine hours a night. According to the National Sleep Foundation, people in the United States now sleep an average of 6.9 hours on weeknights and 7.5 hours on weekends.

A whopping one-third of our population sleeps 6.5 or fewer hours nightly—far less than the 8 hours that many sleep specialists recommend. Physician Will Wilkoff, MD, author of *Is My Child Overtired?*, says the number of overtired patients he sees has soared in the twenty-five years he has been in practice, because families are trying "to squeeze 28 hours of living into 24."

Groundbreaking research is showing that there is a correlation between the lack of sleep so many Americans are experiencing and the weight gain that is plaguing our nation. "We've known that people use food as a pick-me-up when they are tired, but now it appears they are hungrier than we realized, and there is a hormonal basis for their eating," says Thomas Wadden, director of the Weight and Eating Disorders Program at the University of Pennsylvania in Philadelphia.

Columbia University studied the sleep habits of 3,682 people and found that those who got by on less than four hours of sleep a night were 73 percent more likely to be obese than those who slept seven to nine hours nightly. Those catching a modest six hours of sleep a night were 23 percent more likely to be obese. Other studies report that reducing sleep to 6.5 or fewer hours for successive nights causes potentially harmful metabolic, hormonal, and immune changes that can lead to illnesses and diseases such as cancer, diabetes, obesity, and heart disease.

It's plain to see that getting plenty of refreshing sleep on a consistent basis, and enough sleep to meet your body's needs, could be far better for your weight loss goals than eating a diet bar for lunch every day, and just as important as working out and eating right.

THE VALUE OF REFRESHING SLEEP

No one knows exactly why we sleep, but we do know that during the deepest phases of sleep, appetite-regulating hormones are released, energy is restored, the immune system is strengthened, repairs are completed, and healing hormones are released. During REM (rapid-eye-movement) sleep, we have vivid dreams and our brains may be working on consolidating memories. Moreover, a study published in *Nature* found that our brain restructures new memories during sleep, helping us solve problems and become more insightful.

What Is a Good Night's Sleep?

A good night's sleep doesn't simply involve lying on your fluffy pillow for seven to nine hours. The time spent snoozing should also be restful and restorative. Restorative sleep involves sleeping through the night without awakening, or with few awakenings, and also experiencing all the stages of sleep the body was meant to enjoy.

Many people find that not only are they sleeping less these days, but the sleep they do get is not deep and restorative. Nonrestorative sleep (NRS) appears to be the result of modern industrialized society. Because of NRS, more and more people are waking up tired, and they are irritable, lack concentration, are less productive throughout the day, and are hungrier, even when they've slept eight hours.

Sleep is meant to heal and rejuvenate the body physically, mentally, and emotionally. But for a growing number of people, it doesn't. After a night of tossing and turning, waking up frequently, and dreaming fitful dreams, most people are exhausted. Then their day begins, stressors impact their waking hours, and appetite-stimulating hormones pump into their system. Compounding the problem, NRS contributes not only to weight gain but also to such conditions as chronic pain (such as fibromyalgia), muscle aches, heart disease, cancer, chronic fatigue syndrome, immune system dysfunction, and many illnesses, as well as various sleep disorders. Lack of sleep or NRS is also related to safety issues such as car accidents and medical errors, plus impaired job performance and loss of productivity in numerous other activities.

THE STAGES OF SLEEP

Sleep is divided into two states known as non-rapid-eye-movement sleep (NREM) and rapid-eye-movement sleep (REM). These two states occur in a ninety-minute cycle, which is repeated five to six times a night and includes at least four stages of NREM and REM. NREM sleep is the state from which REM sleep emerges. There are altogether five stages of sleep.

Stage 1 sleep. This first sleep stage is experienced as falling to sleep and is a transition stage between being awake and asleep. It usually lasts between one and five minutes and occupies approximately 2 to 5 percent of a normal night of sleep. This stage is dramatically prolonged in some people with insomnia who suffer from restless legs syndrome or disorders that produce frequent arousals such as sleep apnea.

Stage 2 sleep or theta sleep. Theta sleep follows Stage 1 and is the baseline of sleep. This stage is part of the ninety-minute cycle and occupies approximately 45 to 60 percent of the sleep cycle.

Stages 3 and 4 or delta sleep. Stage 2 sleep evolves into delta sleep or slow-wave sleep (SWS) in approximately ten to twenty minutes and may last fifteen to thirty minutes. It's called slow-wave sleep because brain activity slows dramatically from the theta rhythm of Stage 2 to a much slower rhythm of one to two cycles per second called delta; the height or amplitude of the waves increases dramatically as well. In most adults, these two stages are completed within the first two ninety-minute sleep cycles or within the first three hours of sleep. Contrary to popular belief, it is delta sleep (not REM) that is the deepest and most restorative stage of sleep. Delta sleep is what a sleep-deprived person's brain craves most. In children, delta sleep can occupy up to 40 percent of sleep time. This is what makes children difficult to awaken during most of the night.

Stage 5: REM (rapid-eye-movement) sleep. This is a very active stage of sleep. It composes 20 to 25 percent of a normal night's sleep. Breathing, heart rate, and brain wave activity quicken. Vivid dreams often occur. Sleep specialists call this fifth stage of sleep REM because a person's eyes are moving rapidly. After the REM stage, the body usually returns to Stage 2, theta sleep.

HOW MUCH SLEEP DO WE NEED?

Everyone is different. There is no one-size-fits-all when it comes to sleep needs. Though most people need seven to nine hours, some people need as little as four hours while others need ten. The important thing to note is how you function during the day. Are you tired, sleepy, hungry, lacking in concentration, or irritable? If so, perhaps you are not getting enough sleep or you are not sleeping well.

You can determine the amount of sleep your body needs by following these recommendations. Go to bed at the same time each night and see when you naturally wake up without an alarm. Or, if you've been sleep-deprived, the next time you have two consecutive days when you can sleep in—perhaps a weekend or a vacation—sleep as much as you can the first couple of days. That way you can pay your sleep debt. Then, once your sleep has stabilized, record how much you sleep naturally without an alarm, plus or minus fifteen minutes. (You may have to go to bed extra early the third night if you have to get up early for work just to see when you naturally wake up.) That's your sleep need or capacity.

MAKING UP YOUR SLEEP DEFICIT

If you think you can go for a few days with much less sleep than normal and then get a good eight to nine hours, feel rested, and get right back on schedule, you may be disappointed. You'll have to make up your sleep deficit, say the experts. That means you will actually have to sleep the hours you missed to make up the difference.

Does that mean that if you've missed years of sleeping well, you'll have to become Rip Van Winkle—the character in a children's story who slept for twenty years? Not exactly. But while you won't have to hibernate for a year or two, you do need to sleep extra hours for a while. Many people find that at times they need even more make-up sleep than the hours of sleep lost because they're so exhausted. Harvard undergraduates, a high-achieving, sleep-deprived population, frequently go home for Christmas vacation and pretty much sleep for the first week.

Dr. Charles Czeisler, chair of Harvard Medical School's Division of Sleep Medicine, says, "Someone restricted to only five hours of nightly sleep for weeks builds up a cumulative sleep deficit. In the first place, their performance will be as impaired as if they had been up all night. Secondly, it will take two to three weeks of extra nightly sleep before they return to baseline performance. Chronic sleep deprivation's impact takes much longer to build up, and it also takes much longer to recover."

Naps can help you make up a sleep deficit. Short naps, up to forty minutes, can be helpful. Otherwise, you'll go into deep sleep and be groggy when you wake up. If you need more sleep, nap for at least two hours, which will allow your body to slumber through a full ninety-minute sleep cycle and awaken refreshed.

THE LINKS AMONG SLEEP, HORMONES, AND WEIGHT LOSS

A number of studies have found direct links among lack of sleep, the hormones that get out of balance as a result, and weight gain. "Sleep loss disrupts a complex and interwoven series of metabolic and hormonal processes and may be a contributing factor to obesity," says John Winkelman, MD, PhD, medical director of the Sleep Health Center at Brigham and Women's Hospital and assistant professor of psychiatry at Harvard Medical School.

When we don't get adequate sleep, some key hormones get out of whack, namely leptin, ghrelin, cortisol, insulin, and growth hormone.

HORMONES DISRUPTED BY LOSS OF SLEEP

Leptin. The hormone leptin regulates the metabolism of carbohydrates and signals the body when it should feel full and begin making fat; it is significantly affected by lack of sleep. When there are low levels of leptin, the body craves extra food, especially carbohydrates, regardless of whether or not adequate calories have been consumed. This can easily lead to weight gain.

Ghrelin. Ghrelin triggers appetite and has been found at higher levels in those who get too little sleep. It also suppresses fat utilization in fat tissue.

Insulin. The hormone insulin helps manage glucose metabolism. Low insulin levels cause increased appetite, poor sugar metabolism, and hypoglycemia. Continual big spikes and dips in insulin can cause insulin resistance and lead to type 2 diabetes. Low insulin during the night can contribute to low blood sugar, known as nocturnal hypoglycemia, which can cause you to awaken and not get back to sleep.

Cortisol. Cortisol plays a role in regulating appetite. The more balanced your cortisol levels, the easier it is to control your appetite. Too much of this stress hormone, on the other hand, can cause fat deposition, especially around the midsection. And if this hormone is secreted in high amounts during the night, you won't be able to sleep well.

Growth hormone (GH). A lack of sleep can diminish the production of GH—a hormone that helps inhibit weight gain. GH plays an important role in controlling fat deposition and muscle development. Having less of this hormone increases your chances of not sleeping well and being overweight.

When this happens, we can end up with an uncontrollable appetite, and we often crave the most fattening foods. We won't be able to handle stress as well. And our deranged hormones can even cause us to sleep poorly, further compounding the problem.

As you read this book, you'll see just how important it is to sleep the hours your body needs and to sleep well so that you can balance these hormones. In the sections that follow, leptin, a major hormone that controls appetite, is discussed at length because it has such a significant impact on appetite and weight loss. And following leptin, insulin, ghrelin, cortisol, and growth hormone imbalances are covered, because all these hormones are affected when you don't get adequate sleep.

Many people have these hormone imbalances. You may have such imbalances and not even know it. Maybe you tend to crave things you really don't want to eat, or there are times it's harder to lose weight than others. Perhaps there are some days when you handle stress better than others, and days when you don't sleep very well. All these symptoms can be hormone-related.

The good news is that our four-step Sleep Away the Pounds Program will help you bring your hormones into balance. It's all four aspects of the plan—sleep, stress reduction, exercise, and diet—that best help you bring your body into harmony so you can lose weight and enjoy the life you were meant to live.

LEPTIN: THE APPETITE-SUPPRESSING HORMONE

Leptin was discovered in 1994. It is manufactured in the fat cells and communicates to your brain when you should be hungry, eat, and begin fat creation. The name is derived from the Greek word *leptos,* which means "thin". It serves important functions in regulating body weight, metabolism, and reproductive function. Leptin plays a vital role in controlling the brain's hypothalamus activity, which in turn regulates much of the body's autonomic functions—the ones we don't think about, but which determine our health and affect our weight. Just how powerful is leptin in weight management? When leptin was given to mice, it helped reduce fat tissue and boosted insulin sensitivity. Research mice that lack leptin overeat to the point of morbid obesity.

Research conducted at Brown Medical School and Rhode Island Hospital, as well as Harvard Medical School and Beth Israel Deaconess Medical Center, has shown that leptin triggers production of the active form of the peptide AMSH—an appetite suppressant in the hypothalamus, the small area in the base of the brain that controls hunger and metabolism. Researchers say this peptide is one of the body's most powerful metabolism-boosting signals, sending a strong message to the brain to burn calories. This message is then sent to another part of the hypothalamus, where another peptide is released. This stimulates the pituitary gland, which in turn secretes a hormone that relays the message to the thyroid, the master gland of metabolism. Once activated, the thyroid spreads word to the body's cells to increase energy production. And voilà! You're on your way to burning calories and losing weight.

A research team at the University of Chicago reported at the 2001 Association of Professional Sleep Societies meeting in Chicago that in experiments, sleep-deprived volunteers showed leptin changes that promoted weight gain. Men who were allowed only four hours of sleep per night displayed a dip in leptin that was equivalent to that seen in people underfed by a thousand calories a day for three days. In other words, the leptin signal was telling the men's bodies that they were short about a thousand calories. That misleading signal could cue the body to slow metabolism, overstimulate appetite, and increase fat deposition.

LEPTIN PLAYS A PART IN THESE PHYSICAL RESPONSES

- Hunger
- Stress response
- Fat burning and storage
- Body temperature

- Heart rate
- Reproductive behavior
- Bone growth
- Blood sugar levels

Normal leptin levels or increasing leptin levels will not help everyone lose a large amount of weight. For some people, it's simply poor nutrition and lack of exercise that are causing them to tip the scales. But for many, the best diet and exercise program in the world won't work, nor will even the best stress-reduction protocol, unless they develop a good sleep plan, because it's lack of sleep that is causing an imbalance of leptin and the other important hormones that regulate appetite.

Just like everything else, some people are more susceptible to problems with leptin levels than others. Many people who try to lose weight can find it difficult, even if they eat smaller portions than trim people and exercise consistently—all due to problems with leptin, known as leptin resistance.

Leptin Resistance: A Weight Loss Nightmare

Do you often crave sweets, bread, cereal, pasta, crackers, chips, potatoes, soda pop, wine, or beer? Uncontrollable sugar or other carbohydrate cravings, stress eating, hypothyroid symptoms, low energy, and excess abdominal fat can be signs of leptin resistance. If any of these symptoms apply to you, there's a chance you may have developed leptin resistance.

A LANDMARK STUDY LINKING BODY WEIGHT TO SLEEP

In the November 2004 issue of the *Journal of Clinical Endocrinology & Metabolism*, Eve Van Cauter, PhD, and her research team at the Research Laboratory on Sleep, Chronobiology, and Neuroendocrinology at the University of Chicago School of Medicine reported that pre-breakfast concentrations of the satiety hormone leptin were roughly 20 percent lower in healthy men who had slept only four hours a night for nearly a week than when they had slept nine hours nightly. The study involved eleven healthy twenty-two-year-old men who spent consecutive nights in the university's sleep laboratory. For six days, they got only four hours of sleep per night. One year later, the men returned for a six-day study with an eight-hour sleep period, so they served as their own comparison group.

After their six-day sleep-deprivation period, volunteers had a measurable leptin decrease ranging from 19 to 26 percent. This decrease indicated that an erroneous signal was sent by the brain that more food was needed when, in fact, enough food had been eaten. Since the men were getting the same amounts of calories and activity, leptin levels and appetite control should not have changed. In fact, they changed in a major way. The men craved more food and predominantly rich, fattening foods.

In this case, your brain does not detect your body's level of leptin properly and, therefore, does not know how much fat you have in storage. Your brain may think you are the perfect weight and, therefore, not tell your body to burn fat. Worse yet, it can signal that you are short on calories and cause you to want to eat more food, even when that's the last thing you need.

Studies suggest that the tongue is a target for leptin, and that leptin may be a sweet-sensing suppressor that may take part in regulation of food intake, states Dr. Kirio Kawai of Tokyo Medical and Dental University in Japan. In addition to suppressing the appetite, leptin appears to reduce cravings for sweets by targeting taste receptors on the tongue. Therefore, it is possible that a lack of leptin, or the body's failure to respond to this hormone due to defects in leptin receptors (known as leptin resistance), may contribute to the so-called sweet tooth and alcohol and carbohydrate cravings so many people struggle to overcome.

Since leptin is the hormone that controls ghrelin (the hormone that causes us to want to eat), it would seem logical that the more leptin present in the bloodstream, the better. That, however, is not true. When leptin was first discovered, scientists thought they had finally found the answer to obesity. But when they measured leptin levels in overweight people, they found that almost all of them were not leptin-deficient, but in fact had too much of this hormone. It turns out that many of these people were leptin-resistant, meaning they had lost their sensitivity to leptin in the same manner as many people become insulin-resistant, causing a higher level of leptin in their systems. (Leptin and insulin resistance are often at the root of blood sugar imbalance and the overwhelming urge to eat more food.)

Here's how the imbalance works. If you're leptin-resistant, it takes more and more leptin to signal your brain that your body is satisfied and doesn't need to eat more. Ron Rosedale, MD, says it's like people who grow progressively harder of hearing. The bell has to ring louder and louder for them to hear it. Eventually, they won't hear it at all. So it is with leptin resistance—the brain is not receiving leptin's message. Consequently, more and more fat is stored. Here's why. Fat cells make leptin. When people are leptin-resistant, more and more fat cells are perceived as needed to produce more leptin. It's a frustrating cycle. You're hungry because your brain tells you you're not storing enough fat. You eat more food because your brain sends you the signal to eat. The only way to stop eating is to produce more leptin, which means you need more fat—and that causes you to gain more weight. Thus you become more leptin- and insulin-resistant, which makes you keep eating, and eating, and eating.

To top it all off, you more than likely won't be sleeping well. The reason is that leptin resistance causes you to have higher amounts of adrenaline coursing through your body during the night hours when you should be sleeping. (Adrenaline is part of the fight-or-flight chemistry that gets your body going under stress.) So rather than dreaming of dancing sugarplums, you may be awake thinking about eating them. The more sleep-deprived you become, the more intolerant you are of stress. Adding to the fray at this point, even a little stress will elevate the hormone ghrelin, causing you to want to eat more food.

There are several signs that can indicate that you may have a problem with your leptin levels. These include:

- Sleeping less than seven to eight hours per night and feeling tired during the day
- Late-night eating
- Stress eating
- Weight gain around the middle
- Yo-yo dieting
- Low-thyroid symptoms
- Uncontrollable cravings, especially for sugar, alcohol, or simple carbohydrates
- Insomnia or other sleep disorders

This scenario is not counter to how we've been wired, however: We are actually designed for leptin and insulin resistance. It's true. People in times past feasted in summer and early fall when food was plentiful, to store fat for winter when food was scarce. Hence summer was a time to eat as much as possible, and as many carbs as possible (which were probably fruit and honey), so that enough weight could be gained to make it through the winter months. Our survival as a civilization depended on this biochemistry. Today our artificial lights and heat are on in the evening, we stay up late as though it were summer, and we eat carbs just like it was August or September. It's perfectly logical that our bodies think it's summer, causing many of us to become leptin- and insulin-resistant so we can "store fat for winter."

INSULIN AND INSULIN RESISTANCE

Insulin is a hormone secreted by the pancreas that determines whether blood sugar gets used for immediate energy or stored as fat. The body monitors blood sugar levels and cell demands, and releases insulin according to need. Insulin helps cells absorb glucose from the bloodstream by binding with receptors on cells the way a key would fit into a lock. Once the key—insulin—has unlocked the door, the glucose can pass from the blood into the cell. Inside the cell, glucose is either used for energy or stored in the form of glycogen in liver or muscle cells. This process is why a healthy body is described as insulin-sensitive.

Regularly getting too little sleep alters eating behavior and metabolism, says Esra Tasali, MD, a sleep specialist at the University of Chicago. Sleep deprivation has a detrimental impact on insulin sensitivity and carbohydrate metabolism, leaving us at risk of fat gain, especially around the waistline. And when we sleep too little, we produce more cortisol, which in turn causes the release of more insulin. High insulin levels prevent cells from breaking down fat, making it harder to lose weight when dieting. And with a loss of sleep, the body may not be able to metabolize carbohydrates well, which leads to increased storage of fats and higher levels of blood sugar. Excess blood sugar can lead to insulin resistance.

When you eat a lot of refined carbohydrates year after year, a dangerous cascade occurs. Insulin levels remain chronically high, and cells become less responsive and more resistant to insulin. As a consequence, relatively little glucose gets burned, and blood sugar levels remain high. With chronically elevated glucose levels, insulin resistance develops.

Insulin resistance means that the body has trouble disposing of glucose. People who are insulin-resistant have receptor sites that no longer recognize insulin; thus, glucose can't get into the cells. In other words, the key no longer unlocks the door, and the cells are literally starving. As the cells continue to resist insulin, blood sugar levels rise. As a result, the pancreas produces more insulin to help move glucose into the cells, and blood insulin levels go up even higher. Eventually, the pancreas can no longer produce enough insulin to compensate for the insulin resistance, causing blood glucose levels to rise more and more and diabetes to develop. (People with insulin resistance—with or without the presence of diabetes—are predisposed to heart disease and abnormal accumulation and elevation of triglycerides and cholesterol. There is also some evidence that it may contribute to endometrial cancer and Alzheimer's disease.)

Sleep plays a key role in insulin resistance. From sleep-restriction experiments, it's clear that after just a week of sleep loss, insulin levels are higher and the ability to use blood sugar is dramatically altered. A study published in the *Lancet* in October 1999 clearly demonstrated the relationships among sleep, overeating, impaired glucose metabolism, and insulin resistance. Eve Van Cauter, PhD, and her associates studied eleven healthy, normal-weight young men for two weeks in a sleep lab. In just one week, the researchers observed that sleep deficits of several hours a night actually impaired the body's processing of glucose, and the young men showed signs of insulin resistance. In a follow-up study, short sleepers showed 50 percent more insulin resistance than did the controls. Dr. Van Cauter said that reduced sleep could accelerate the onset of diabetes, which can be due to the imbalance in blood sugar and resistance to insulin.

YOU CAN REVERSE LEPTIN AND INSULIN RESISTANCE

To halt the cycle of insulin and leptin resistance, you'll need to retrain your brain and your cells. Lifestyle changes as outlined below can correct this resistance and restore balance to your body. As you follow our plan, you should be on your way to correcting insulin and leptin resistance quickly and losing weight as a result.

The Sleep Away the Pounds Program incorporates adequate sleep, exercise, weight management, and dietary changes. This helps your body respond more effectively to insulin and leptin. By getting the sleep you need, avoiding various foods and eating plenty of the recommended foods, losing weight, and being more physically active, you can improve insulin and leptin sensitivity. This may help you avoid type 2 diabetes and other serious illnesses in the future. In fact, a major study has verified the benefits of healthy lifestyle changes, blood glucose management, and weight loss. In 2001, the National Institutes of Health completed the Diabetes Prevention Program (DPP), a clinical trial designed to find the most effective ways of preventing type 2 diabetes in overweight people with pre-diabetes. The researchers found that lifestyle changes reduced the risk of diabetes by 58 percent. And many people with pre-diabetes returned to normal blood glucose levels.

Here are some specific things you can do right away to reach your goal of becoming insulin- and leptin-sensitive and managing your blood glucose levels. Start by regularly getting seven to nine hours of sleep or the number of hours of sleep your body needs. And make sure your sleep is refreshing and restorative. You'll know this is occurring when you wake up refreshed and energized every day.

Incorporate regular physical activity into your schedule. Exercise helps your muscle cells use blood glucose for energy. It enhances your body's ability to utilize glucose more effectively, and it increases the number of insulin receptor sites on each cell's surface. It also normalizes leptin levels. Studies investigating long-duration exercise (an hour or more) indicate that serum leptin concentrations are reduced with such exercise. (A reduction in serum leptin levels can indicate that cells are utilizing leptin more efficiently, providing that you are meeting your sleep needs as well. Otherwise, lower leptin levels could be the result of sleep deprivation.)

Weight loss is also a key. Plasma leptin and insulin concentrations are tightly coupled with fat mass, so decreases in fat cells due to weight loss coincide with decreased concentrations of circulating leptin and insulin. Several studies suggest that a weight loss as modest as ten pounds can decrease blood glucose levels, which makes the cells more receptive to insulin and leptin, thereby decreasing insulin and leptin resistance.

Dietary changes focus on avoiding the foods that cause surges in leptin and insulin production. Insulin and leptin resistance is caused in large part by the overconsumption of refined carbohydrates, such as breads, pastas, alcohol, and sugary foods, and by eating too much fat, which includes saturated fat as found in animal products, trans fats as found in margarine, fried foods, and snack foods, and the omega-6 fatty acids found in vegetable oils. Make special effort to avoid sweets, sodas, and alcohol; refined carbohydrates such as breads, pasta, white rice, and pizza; and polyunsaturated oils like corn, soy, sunflower, and safflower. Also, limit animal products high in saturated fat. Note, too, that eating too *little* essential fatty acid contributes to the resistance problem. It is important to increase foods rich in omega-3 fatty acids such as fish (especially salmon, mackerel, and trout), fish oils such as cod-liver oil, and leafy green vegetables, along with nuts, especially walnuts, and seeds—flax seeds in particular. Increase brightly colored vegetables, low-sugar fruit, and beans. Avoid all sugar substitutes, fake fats, and artificial flavors. You may choose foods containing these substitutes to reduce caloric intake, but these foods can cause pronounced food cravings and an uncontrollable appetite, causing you to eat much more than normal while leaving your body nutrient-depleted. Such substitutes have been associated in studies with weight gain rather than weight loss.

GHRELIN: THE APPETITE-STIMULATING HORMONE

In the last few years, research has begun pointing to an array of diet and lifestyle factors (sleep deprivation is one of the primary ones) that modify the body's production of the hormone ghrelin—the appetite-stimulating hormone that gives people the munchies. Researchers have found that a spike in ghrelin after a short night of sleep can lead to indiscriminate and sometimes out-of-control eating patterns. For example, a sleep study conducted by Dr. Van Cauter found that individuals with the biggest hormonal changes craved the most fattening foods, including ice cream, cakes, candy, pasta, bread, and salty snacks such as potato chips. There were no cravings for fruits and vegetables.

Dubbed ghrelin, after a Hindu word for "growth," this twenty-eight-amino-acid peptide reflects a complex interplay of chemical signals that scientists are now beginning to unravel. Ghrelin was discovered as the peptide hormone that potently stimulates the release of growth hormone from the anterior pituitary gland. It was determined that ghrelin, along with several other hormones, has significant appetite-stimulating effects.

Secreted by epithelial cells in the stomach and the upper part of the small intestine, ghrelin acts on the brain. In both rodents and humans, ghrelin increases hunger through its action on the hypothalamic feeding centers. Humans injected with ghrelin reported sensations of intense hunger; in one study, when turned loose at a buffet, they ate 30 percent more food than they would normally.

Ghrelin appears to suppress fat utilization in adipose (fat) tissue. This may explain why dieters who lose weight and then try to keep it off make more ghrelin than they did before dieting. It's as if their bodies are fighting to regain the lost fat, researchers reported in the *New England Journal of Medicine.* In short, their bodies seem to be trying to hold on to fat stores in case there is another "famine."

The featured players in appetite suppression and ghrelin management include insulin, which is made in the pancreas (a lack of insulin increases a rodent's call to eat), and leptin, manufactured by fat cells. These two hormones turn down the dial on ghrelin production and help control appetite when your diet is high on plenty of refreshing sleep.

CORTISOL: THE HORMONE THAT AFFECTS METABOLISM AND BELLY FAT

Sleep loss affects the hormones of the hypothalamic-pituitary-adrenal (HPA) axis. In a natural rhythm with the sleep–wake cycle, cortisol, one of these HPA axis hormones, is released at various times throughout the day and night. It is commonly released in response to physical or emotional stress, in effect prolonging the body's fight-or-flight response. When we are deprived of sleep, cortisol is released at an increased level, which makes us feel hungry even if we're full. As a result, people who continue to lose sleep on a regular basis will tend to experience hunger even when they have had an adequate amount of food.

Cortisol also raises blood sugar and insulin levels, which causes an increase in fat deposition, especially on the belly. The increase in blood sugar then stimulates a further increase in insulin, which sets off a whole scenario of problems discussed earlier. In addition, it causes fluid retention, muscle weakness, memory loss, and high blood pressure. It also has detrimental effects on other aspects of our endocrine system, such as thyroid gland function, which governs our metabolism. (A slow metabolism causes us to gain weight.)

According to a study published in the *Lancet*, sleep deprivation causes an elevation of stress hormone levels in the evening as well as a heightened stress response throughout the day. Normally, levels of cortisol should decrease at night, increase as morning approaches, and peak around the time the sun rises as part of the body's physiological response to awakening, preparing it to face the day alert and energized. Without realizing it, some people are stuck in a hyperalert state all night with cortisol levels high throughout the night; consequently, they sleep lightly or awaken constantly. Others are "off cycle," with cortisol peaking in the night followed by low cortisol levels in the morning. These people often awaken during the night and are unable to return to sleep, sometimes for hours, if at all, and are tired and groggy in the morning and hungry throughout the day.

Oversecretion or a disrupted secretion of cortisol can drastically interfere with slow-wave delta sleep, which occurs primarily when cortisol levels are decreasing. Wakefulness and Stage 1 sleep are associated with increased plasma cortisol concentrations, which are meant to rise only in the morning. When cortisol is out of balance, it can contribute to insomnia and also the tendency to awaken often during the night, and to feel unrefreshed even after getting a full night's sleep.

Adequate and refreshing sleep effectively reduces cortisol. When hormones such as cortisol are balanced and secreted in the proper cycle, we should sleep well all night and awaken refreshed and restored physically, mentally, and emotionally.

GROWTH HORMONE, FAT BURNING, AND MUSCLE DEVELOPMENT

Growth hormone (GH), a microscopic protein substance, is produced in the anterior section of the pituitary gland deep in the brain. It is a tissue-building hormone that causes growth, enacts repairs, mobilizes fat stores, and shifts the metabolism into high gear in the presence of amino acids. Chemically, it is somewhat similar to insulin, and is secreted in short pulses during the first hours of sleep and after exercise, but it remains in circulation for only a few minutes. The body binds most of the GH in the liver and converts some of it into another protein hormone called insulin-like growth factor 1 (IGF-1). Although IGF-1 is not insulin, it acts like insulin as it promotes glucose transfer through cell membranes into the cell. More important, IGF-1 elicits most of the effects associated with GH.

GH is responsible for the development of lean body mass, bone density, and an efficient metabolism that diminishes the body's fat-storing capacity. During deep sleep, there is an increased secretion of GH. This is necessary for repairing and rebuilding body tissues such as muscle and bone. It also helps combat the negative effects of cortisol. Losing sleep, especially deep sleep, decreases GH levels. Since GH helps regulate the body's proportions of fat and muscle, less GH reduces our ability to lose fat and develop muscle. Muscle development is important for weight loss in that it is responsible for burning more calories, even at a resting heart rate. (Be aware that if a woman is testosterone-deficient, she will not be able to build muscle mass no matter how much she works out. Testosterone production relies on adequate levels of the hormone progesterone, as well as of cholesterol.)

GH secretion follows a circadian rhythm and occurs in six to twelve pulses per day, with the largest pulse secreted about an hour or two after the onset of deep sleep—Stages 3 and 4. If we don't get to the deep-sleep stage, we end up sabotaging our body's capacity to repair and renew tissues and cells. And unless we get to that sound-sleep zone, our bodies will not be releasing GH efficiently. This can be a frustrating scenario because low GH can *cause* people to be light sleepers.

GH has been shown to decline with age, but now some scientists say age is not the factor that inhibits the body's release of GH. It's the physiological changes that accompany aging that are responsible for it—changes such as weight gain, obesity, high blood sugar levels, and high levels of free fatty acids in the blood. All these factors are to a large extent controllable by getting adequate sleep, nutrition, and exercise—which means that there is a lot we can do now to stimulate the body's release of GH. For example, a workout that is strenuous enough to create muscle exhaustion releases GH. The exercise must be at the right level of intensity—not so high that it causes injury and suppresses the body's release of the hormone (marathoners, for example, show decreased levels of GH), yet strong and resistant enough to bring about fat loss and metabolic efficiency. When muscles contract and relax during multiple sets of resistance exercises, the body is stimulated to produce significant levels of GH to repair and renew the tissues. The diet recommended for reversing insulin and leptin resistance is also the diet that is key to improving release of GH. And getting adequate, deep sleep is imperative, which the entire Sleep Away the Pounds Program is dedicated to helping you achieve.

SLEEP: A MISSING LINK
TO WEIGHT LOSS

Beyond your being bleary-eyed, clutching a latte, and dozing off at afternoon meetings, failing to get enough sleep or sleeping at odd hours heightens your chance for weight gain and a variety of illnesses.

Now that you know about the sleep research and how a loss of sleep can give you a major case of the munchies, why not try a little experiment? The next time you have to be up late or get up extra early, and you end up sleep-deprived by a few hours, take note of your appetite. Do you want to eat more food? What foods do you choose? Are you ready to grab the first bag of chips or candy bar in sight? We think you'll be amazed as you discover just how much sleep affects your appetite.

In the following chapter, you will be presented with the tools you need to revamp your nightlife so you can get your best sleep, starting today. This is the first and most important step in your weight loss plan. Learning and exploring these relatively simple techniques is your ticket to a slimmer you.

Chapter Two

Step One: Your Best Sleep Now

While many aspects of sleep are a mystery—including exactly why we sleep—the picture emerging from current research is that not sleeping enough or being awake in the wee hours runs counter to the body's internal clock, throwing a host of basic bodily functions out of sync. Physiological studies suggest that a sleep deficit may put our bodies into a state of high alert, increasing the production of stress- and appetite-inducing hormones, driving up blood pressure, and causing us to want to eat more food, often rich, fattening fare.

Sleep loss increases the activity of the vagus nerve, which sends signals between the gut and the brain. During sleep deprivation, the brain signals the body to release appetite-stimulating hormones such as ghrelin, and to suppress appetite-controlling hormones such as leptin, which appears to be the mechanism by which sleep loss and other forms of stress change eating behavior.

There may be a good reason for this hormonal alteration. In the days before artificial lights and stimulants, when people had to be up in the middle of the night, it was most likely in order to gather food or escape danger. At such times, more fuel was needed. Perhaps the body is naturally wired for appetite-stimulating hormones to be released when we're up late.

It's easy to see that when we're short on sleep, our bodies may actually be craving a bed and a pillow. That's a hunger only sleep can satisfy, though we may try to fill it with lots of food. When you find yourself craving various foods, are you actually hungry for a night of refreshing sleep? It is possible that the right amount of sleep for you on a consistent basis has been the missing component in your weight loss efforts.

Poor sleep habits are among the most common problems we encounter in Western society. We stay up too late, get up too early, and cross time zones frequently, disrupting our circadian rhythms (the natural twenty-four-hour sleep–wake cycle). We interrupt sleep with drugs, chemicals, parties, and work. We overeat and drink at night. And we overstimulate our bodies with caffeine, and our minds with television and computers. No wonder our bodies are out of whack and overweight.

You may be getting the recommended seven to nine hours of sleep a night, but are you truly resting? By brushing up on what sleep specialists refer to as your sleep hygiene (hygiene is the science that deals with the preservation of health), you can help make each night a truly rejuvenating experience that balances the biochemistry of your body for optimum functioning and jump-starts weight loss. With the more than sixty practical tips in this chapter, you can be on your way to making Step One of the Sleep Away the Pounds Program—getting your best sleep possible each night—an integral part of your weight loss plan.

PRACTICAL TIPS TO HELP YOU GET A GOOD NIGHT'S SLEEP

The following sleep tips can help you achieve your best sleep possible so you can maximize your weight loss.

Go to sleep at the same time each night and get up at the same time each morning. This will establish a routine where your body becomes used to falling asleep at a specific time.

Go to bed as early as possible, but no later than 10 PM. "Studies suggest that if you normally need eight hours of sleep and you get them between 10 PM and 6 AM, you'll feel more rested than if you go to sleep at midnight and get up at 8 AM," says David Simon, MD, medical director of the Chopra Center in La Jolla, California. Your entire body, but particularly your adrenal glands, does the majority of its recharging or recovering between 11 PM and 1 AM, says Dr. Joseph Mercola. In addition, your gallbladder dumps toxins during this same period. Mercola adds that if you are awake, the toxins back up into your liver, which then secondarily backs up into your entire system, causing further disruption of your health. Prior to the widespread use of electricity, people would go to bed shortly after sundown.

During winter, it's best to go to bed around 9 PM. It is quite possible that our bodies are wired for more sleep during the darker days of winter. When we're up late with artificial lights at night during winter months, we may be sending a message that it's summer and time to load up on calories, particularly carbs, for the coming winter fast when typically food was scarce in days of yore.

Avoid lengthy napping in the middle of the day. To keep on track, avoid taking long naps—more than forty minutes—or late-afternoon naps. Limit your naptime to fifteen to forty minutes, about eight hours after you wake up. Napping does appear to be part of our ancestral heritage and is part of the natural sleep–wake cycle.

Avoid caffeine and nicotine, especially late in the day. Caffeine and nicotine are stimulants that can make you jittery and keep you from falling asleep. Caffeine has a half-life of 7.5 hours, meaning that it's still in your bloodstream more than seven hours after eating or drinking it. For some people, caffeine can stay in the body as long as fourteen hours. So be aware that your afternoon latte may be causing some late-night frustration when it comes to getting restful sleep. For some people who are very sensitive, even decaf coffee can have this effect. Also, caffeine can increase the number of awakenings we experience throughout the night.

Avoid alcohol. Though you may feel like nodding off after you have a drink or two, once the effects of alcohol wear off, sleep actually becomes more fitful. Alcohol will also keep you from moving into the deeper stages of sleep, when the body does most of its healing. Many people have a drink to relax, and though alcohol is a sedative, it can have the reverse effect during the night. The alcohol you drink in the evening is metabolized and cleared from your system as you sleep, and can lead to periods of disruption lasting as long as two to three hours. During these periods, your sleep is not as restorative as normal, and you will not feel as rested and refreshed in the morning.

Avoid sugars and refined carbohydrates. These foods have a stimulatory effect and can keep you awake at night. They are also major contributors to a dysfunctional endocrine system, especially adding stress to the adrenal glands, which can cause hormones such as cortisol to get out of whack and totally disrupt your sleep. They are also very fattening foods.

Avoid eating a heavy meal late in the day. Eating a large meal late in the day means the body won't be able to rest later on when it's still trying to digest all that food. Research shows that the timing and size of our evening meal are closely related to how we eat during the day. For instance, when we grab a mug of coffee and a breakfast bar on the way to work, eat a sandwich or a burger and fries for lunch on the run, or put off dinner for a multitude of chores after work, we usually are so starved that we overeat when we do start dinner. We are then setting ourselves up for a bad night's sleep. This practice also contributes significantly to weight gain because eating large meals at night gives the body little chance to burn up calories before going to bed. Your best weight loss and sleep plan is to eat the majority of your food during the day, then have a light dinner.

Eat a light snack before bedtime; this can stabilize your blood sugar. Do not go to bed on an empty stomach if you tend toward low blood sugar (hypoglycemia). Low blood sugar causes the release of hormones that can keep you awake; it's your body's way of saying, *Pssst . . . go find some food, 'cause we're running low here!* Have a light snack of no more than a couple hundred calories. A slice of turkey or some almonds would be good, or have some raw vegetables with a little almond butter. Don't eat too much protein, though, since excess protein can interfere with the entry into the brain of L-tryptophan, an amino acid used to make sleep-inducing serotonin.

Avoid bedtime snacks with sugars and refined carbohydrates. That bowl of ice cream you've come to enjoy at night could be the culprit keeping you awake or making your sleep nonrefreshing. Sugars and refined carbs raise blood sugar and disrupt sleep. (Refined carbs turn to sugar quickly in the bloodstream. See Chapter 8 for information on high-glycemic foods.) Later, when blood sugar drops too low (hypoglycemia), you could wake up and not be able to fall back asleep.

Improve digestion—physical, emotional, and mental. On the physical level, indigestion is caused either by bad food or by impaired digestion and leads to conditions such as heartburn (a contributor to insomnia), flatulence, constipation, and diarrhea. Mental indigestion is the inability to let go of a certain incident or thought—usually an unpleasant experience. Emotional indigestion is the recurrence of a feeling, often sadness or anger, long after the precipitating event. The emotion has not been sufficiently digested and remains just under the surface, springing up for no apparent reason. Mental and emotional indigestion are among the most common causes of disturbed sleep. Some of us even grind our teeth while we sleep, which is often due to stress—usually mental or emotional stress—and is related to an inability to let go.

Drink chamomile tea. Chamomile has a calming, soothing effect on the body and is a traditional sleep-inducing remedy. Swapping a mug of chamomile tea for black tea or coffee after dinner can help improve the quality and quantity of your slumber.

Eat lettuce. Lettuce contains a substance that helps promote sleep by sedating the nervous system. A crisp green salad with supper is a good option to help you drift off to sleep easily. A glass of veggie juice that includes lettuce as an ingredient could be an excellent nightcap.

Take magnesium and calcium supplements. When your calcium or magnesium is too low, you can wake up in the night and not be able to go back to sleep. An article in the *Townsend Letter for Doctors and Patients* by Melvyn R. Werbach noted that "a high magnesium, low aluminum diet has been found to be associated with high-quality sleep time and few nighttime awakenings, and magnesium supplementation has been reported to reduce sleep latency and result in uninterrupted sleep." Magnesium supplementation has also been found to be effective therapy for restless legs syndrome. Magnesium has a sedating effect on the nervous system, and it's one of the nutrients frequently deficient in the American diet. The supplement recommendation is 400 mg of magnesium citrate before bed with a small amount (two to four ounces) of acid-rich juice such as tomato or apple to facilitate absorption. Eat plenty of magnesium-rich foods throughout the day, too, such as leafy green vegetables, avocado, coconut, brown rice, beans, garlic, seeds, and nuts. Focus especially on vegetables rich in magnesium, which include beets, broccoli, cauliflower, carrots, celery, asparagus, green peppers, and winter squash.

Consider a heavy metals detox program if you experience frequent nighttime awakenings. There is some indication that heavy metals such as aluminum, mercury, and cadmium can cause nighttime awakenings.

Make your bedroom temperature cool and comfortable. Be sure that your bedroom is not too warm or too cold during the night. Set your thermostat to a comfortable temperature; experts suggest somewhere between sixty and sixty-five degrees Fahrenheit, but no more than seventy for optimum sleep. A study published in the journal *Sleep* found that a drop in temperature near bedtime causes the body to sense that it's time to go to sleep. A cooler temperature can also help you sleep more restfully. And though they may be comfy when you drift off to sleep, too many blankets or comforters can take your body temperature too high and keep you from deep sleep. (Your body temperature rises naturally during the night.)

Keep your feet warm. Wear socks to bed if your feet get cold. The feet often feel cold before the rest of your body does, making it hard to drift off to sleep. A study has shown that warming your feet reduces nighttime awakenings. If you get too hot in the night, just pull the socks off.

Wiggle your toes. Once you're in bed, lie on your back and wiggle your toes up and down twelve times, wiggling the toes of both feet at the same time. This will help relax your entire body. According to reflexology (foot massage or acupressure applied to certain parts of the feet to promote healing), your feet are like a master control panel for the rest of your body. The ends of meridians (pathways in the body along which energy is believed to flow) in your feet connect with every organ and every part of your body. Toe wiggling helps bring about relaxing, free-flowing energy.

Sniff lavender at bedtime. Dabbing a couple of drops of lavender oil on your temples or on your pillow may help your body relax. Or you can purchase a lavender oil inhaler or aromatherapy diffuser.

Rub your tummy. Tummy rubbing soothes the digestive system and helps bring about deeper relaxation. An extra benefit is that it will help you lose weight by improving digestion. Simply lie on your back and place your hand on your navel. Begin by making small circles in a clockwise direction as you gently glide your hand over your stomach. Gradually make the circles larger and larger. When your circles reach the outside of your stomach, gradually reduce their size until you are back at your navel again. Then reverse the direction to counterclockwise and repeat. Repeat this series with your other hand.

Try deep-breathing exercises. If you have trouble getting to sleep, try the following: Lie on your back and relax your body. Inhale, filling your lower belly, then your stomach, your chest, and finally the top of your lungs with air. Hold for a second or two and exhale slowly. Empty the air to the bottom of your lungs, chest, stomach, and lower belly. Continue this process for several minutes. Don't force your breathing. Just breathe in a relaxed, peaceful mode. While you breathe, imagine that you are resting on a warm ocean beach or floating on a rubber raft in a warm pool with the water rocking you to sleep and the sun shining on your body. Continue breathing until you fall asleep.

Clasp your left thumb with your right hand and place it on your belly. The thumb is thought to represent safety and security, like a little child feels when sucking his thumb. If, after a while, you don't go to sleep, move on to the next finger, and then the next, and so on. Most people don't make it past the third finger.

Release all positional tension. A jerk, startle, or a feeling like you are falling when you are almost asleep lets you know where you are holding tension. Simply remind yourself that the jerk means you are starting to fall asleep, and with that reassurance, release any positional tension (meaning the spot that is tense) and ease into sleep.

Stare at one spot on the ceiling or wall, with your eyes looking up. Your eyelids should become heavy and tired and begin to close, making it easier to drift off to sleep.

Relive a pleasant sleep memory. Use at least three of your senses such as touch, sound, and smell to recall a pleasant memory about your sleep. For example, it may be after a bath when the bed felt particularly comfortable as you drifted off to sleep, or falling asleep curled up in a chair in front of a fireplace, or napping as a passenger in a car, or drifting to sleep under the shade of an umbrella. Whatever it is, relive the sleepy part of the memory to take you off to slumberland.

Try relaxing visualizations. Lie on your back with your eyes closed and imagine you're in your favorite peaceful spot. It may be floating in a swimming pool, lying on a sunny beach, resting on a blanket in a meadow, or dozing in a hammock by a stream. Wherever it is, feel the peaceful sensations—the birds singing, the smell of fragrant flowers, the warmth of the sun, a slight breeze on your cheek, whatever pleases you. Relax. Let go. And drift off to sleep. Return here often. The more you associate this place with falling asleep, the more effective it will become.

Keep your room dark. It's complete darkness that causes your pineal gland to release melatonin, the hormone that promotes sleep. There are light-sensitive monitors built into our eyes, skin, blood, and bone cells. A study at the University of Chicago proved that shining a light from a fiber-optic tube behind the knee of a subject who was completely covered stopped melatonin production. This showed that skin cells can read light and send the message to the pineal gland that it's morning and time to stop producing melatonin. Even the tiniest bit of light in the room can disrupt your circadian rhythm and your pineal gland's production of melatonin and serotonin. There should also be as little light in the bathroom as possible if you get up in the middle of the night. Cover all blinking lights, illuminated clocks, and any other lights in your room. Put up good blinds or drapes that block out all light if you have streetlights outside your window; if this is not possible, wear a sleep mask. Sleeping in complete darkness and experiencing bright light exposure in the daytime is a powerful, natural method to increase your melatonin levels. (It will also help decrease your risk of cancer.)

Get a massage. Get a professional massage, or have someone give you one just before going to sleep. A full-body massage is very relaxing, but if that's not possible, even a short back rub or face-and-scalp massage can be a big help. The massage strokes should be slow, gentle, yet firm, to work the tension out of your muscles and soothe you to sleep.

Rose-colored glasses aren't just for Pollyannas. In a clinical trial, it was found that simply wearing rose-colored glasses after sundown increased melatonin secretion by 70 percent. Pulsing light from a TV or computer screen after dusk wears down melatonin production, while rosy glasses block out light. So if you're going to a movie, watching TV, or staring at a computer in the evening, don't forget your pink-tinted lenses.

Keep the lights in your home low in the evening. Soft lights can help your body wind down and get ready for sleep. Bright lights make your body think it's morning. Consider installing a dimmer switch on your lights so you can turn them down gradually in the evening.

Relax and wind down at least an hour before sleep. Find a relaxing bedtime routine and stick with it. This could be something as simple as reading a book—a really boring book is almost guaranteed to put you to sleep fast. Listening to relaxing music, taking a bath, meditating, or praying can all be helpful, too, in winding down at the end of the day.

Read or do something that is not overly stimulating once you're in bed until you feel sleepy, especially if you can't fall asleep and don't feel drowsy.

Take a warm bath, shower, or sauna before bedtime. When your body temperature is raised in the late evening, it will fall at bedtime, facilitating sleep.

Listen to soft, relaxing music. Soft, soothing music can help lull you to sleep. In a study published in the *Journal of Advanced Nursing*, a team from Taiwan's Tzu Chi University examined the sleep patterns of sixty people, ages sixty through eighty-three, who had difficulty sleeping. Half were given relaxing music to listen to for forty-five minutes at bedtime, and half were given no help to sleep. The team found that those who listened to a selection of soft, relaxing music experienced physical changes that aided restful sleep, such as lower heart and respiratory rates. There are cassettes and CDs designed for this very purpose; some are music specifically composed for sleep, while others have sounds of waves rhythmically breaking or the steady pattern of a heartbeat. Make sure you have a cassette or CD player that turns off automatically; getting up to turn off the player could perk you up.

Sleep on your back. The back is the best position for relaxing, and allows all your internal organs to rest well. Experts recommend that we never sleep on our stomach. It causes pressure on all our internal organs—including the lungs—which causes shallow breathing and can also cause a stiff neck and back problems.

Count cuddly little lambs. Why not try this old remedy for sleep? But make those lambs sleepy, not like many TV commercials that show bouncy, active sheep that make you want to get up and jump around. Your lambs should be drowsy creatures. Imagine a beautiful green meadow stretching out before you. Every few feet or so lies a peaceful, sleeping lamb. Imagine that you're gliding by. You pass a dozing lamb every three or four seconds. Count the lamb and glide on to the next, and the next, and so on, until you've drifted on to sleepland.

Avoid any stimulating activity close to bedtime such as watching TV, Internet or computer work, housework, or arguing. TV, especially, is too stimulating to the brain; it takes longer to fall asleep after watching television, especially something action-packed. It also disrupts your pineal gland function due to the light.

Avoid using your bed for anything other than sleep or sex. It is important that your brain associate your bed with sleeping.

Keep the noise out. Use earplugs if you sleep with a snorer. Also, get the snorer to use one of the nasal sprays to curb snoring; they work quite well. If you live on or near a loud street, running a fan for its white noise may help, in addition to earplugs. And if Fido or Fluffy is restless at night, a dog or cat bed on the floor next to your bed (or maybe down the hall) might be in order.

Listen to relaxation CDs. Some people find nature sounds, such as ocean waves or forest wildlife, to be soothing and helpful in shutting out disturbances like snoring or street noise.

Make a to-do list before you go to bed if you have trouble shutting your mind down when the lights go out. If you continue to worry about things left undone or deadlines for that week, write it all down, including dates and times when you'll get it done. This may help you let go of the worries at night, knowing you'll tackle the list the next day.

Avoid loud alarm clocks. It is very stressful on the body to be jolted out of slumber suddenly. It's much more natural to awaken gradually to the strains of restful music, singing birds, or the jingle of bells. There are also clocks with lights that gradually grow brighter, just like the steady rise of the sun.

Journal. If you often lie in bed with your mind racing about ideas, hobbies, or projects, it might be helpful to keep a journal and write down your thoughts before bed or when you awaken in the night. This tool can help you clear your mind and get to sleep.

Rid your bedroom of electromagnetic fields (EMFs). EMFs can disrupt the pineal gland and the production of melatonin and serotonin, and may have other negative effects on your health.

Unplug lamps, clocks, the TV, the computer, or anything else electric in your bedroom before you go to sleep. If you must use an electric alarm clock, keep it at least three feet from your body. Never sleep with an electric blanket.

Reduce or avoid as many drugs as possible. Many medications, both prescription and over-the-counter, can cause problems with sleep. If you suspect that a medication you are taking is keeping you awake, talk with your doctor or pharmacist about alternatives that won't interfere with your sleep.

If you can't sleep, get out of bed after lying awake for twenty-five minutes and do something calming, such as meditating, reading, praying, or listening to a tape. Do not stay in bed awake for hours, tossing and turning, attempting to will yourself back to sleep. After relaxing out of bed for a short while, get back in bed, again arising after twenty-five minutes if you have not yet fallen asleep. Though this technique is difficult at first, your brain will eventually begin to associate the bed with sleep only. The ultimate goal of this exercise is to send one simple message to your brain—*When in bed, it's time to sleep.*

Lose weight. Being overweight can increase the risk of sleep apnea, which will prevent a restful night's sleep. Obviously, you bought this book so you could lose weight. You're on the right track.

Avoid foods to which you are sensitive or allergic. This is particularly true for dairy and wheat sensitivities, which can cause sleep apnea, excess congestion, and fitful sleep.

Limit your fluids before going to bed. This will reduce your need to get up and go to the bathroom during the night—or at least minimize the frequency.

Remove the clock from view if viewing the time makes you anxious. Constantly staring at 2 AM, 3:30 AM, and 4:15 AM can add to your anxiety about not sleeping. If it does, place your clock where you can't see it.

Choose a comfy mattress. Make sure your mattress is neither too firm nor too soft for you. You want a comfy mattress that's just right for you so your body can relax, you won't toss and turn all night, and your back won't ache in the morning. This is one investment that is truly worth it. If you find that chemicals from your mattress affect your sleep and health, you may want to consider investing in an organic mattress. Though they are more expensive, many owners attest that they're worth the extra cost.

Consider organic cotton bedding. Permanent-press bedding can give off low-grade chemical fumes while you sleep. Your body can deplete nutrients such as zinc and magnesium trying to detoxify chemicals like these. Also, consider not using a fabric sheet in your dryer, which adds more chemicals to your bedding.

Choose a pillow that is comfortable for you. For many people, a pillow that is too thick and raises the head too high can contribute to a stiff neck in the morning and restless sleep at night. If you travel a lot, invest in a small pillow that you can roll up in your suitcase; hotel pillows are often very thick and uncomfortable.

Point your head north or east when you sleep. Feng shui suggests that to help you align your body with the magnetic fields of the earth and bring your own energies into harmony with those of the planet, your head should point north or east. (Feng shui is the Chinese system that studies people's relationships to their environment, particularly their homes, and attempts to achieve maximum physical harmony.) This system also suggests that you never point your head or your feet toward the door, though you should be able to see the door. Placing the bed diagonally in the room is excellent if you have the space.

Choose bedroom colors that are soft and relaxing. Vibrant colors such as red or rose are energizing and can be too stimulating. It is best to choose paint and fabrics that are soft and soothing.

Choose fabrics to sleep in that are cozy and comfortable. Avoid anything that is binding or uncomfortable or fabrics that are too thick and cause you to overheat during the night. Natural fabrics are best—cotton or lightweight flannel, for instance.

Avoid keeping exercise equipment in the bedroom. Exercise equipment connotes active energy, and is best kept somewhere other than the bedroom—or at least keep it covered at night.

Expose your body to bright light or sunlight soon after awakening. This will help regulate your natural biological clock.

Take time out for relaxation and enjoyable experiences. Relaxation and enjoyable experiences help your body heal and promote deep, restful sleep, especially when they involve getting some fresh air.

Prevent jet lag. When traveling, stay hydrated and well nourished, and try to get in sync with the new time zone as soon as possible. In other words, if you arrive in the morning following a red-eye flight to a new time zone, do your best to stay awake all day and go to bed after dark in your new location.

Get regular exercise. Exercising for at least thirty minutes every day can help you fall asleep more easily and stay asleep all night. Working out can reduce stress hormones and increase the time your body spends in deep sleep. Studies show that exercising in the morning is the best if you can do it; otherwise, do avoid anything too strenuous (such as aerobic activity) within three hours of bedtime. This may energize you too much and make it hard to fall asleep.

YOUR SLEEP PRESCRIPTION

- Starting tonight, increase your sleep by thirty minutes. Research shows that even thirty minutes of additional sleep can make a significant difference in your weight loss.
- Determine how much sleep your body needs. See page 8 for how to determine your sleep needs.
- Get the recommended seven to nine hours of sleep each night, unless you need more or less.
- Practice relaxation and stress-reduction techniques and other recommendations in the Sleep Away the Pounds Program to quiet your mind and body so you can get peaceful, restorative sleep. See Chapter 3 for more information.

CHAPTER THREE

Step Two: Quieting the Mind, Restoring the Soul

Too much to do and too little time to do it. Sound familiar? How many times have you been going full speed in the evening hours, trying to get it all done before the next day begins? Frazzled, exhausted, you crawl into bed with your mind still at the computer or poring over the to-do list for the week, your body as alert as a night watchman's.

From time to time, we've all experienced a frantic, stressful lifestyle—and for some of us, it's the norm. With thoughts whirling around in our heads like a high-speed Internet connection, a sheep couldn't possibly get in there to be counted. And we're supposed to fall asleep on cue! There's no way sleep comes easily as we toss and turn with our minds speeding down the information superhighway.

Or we may fall asleep easily but wake up early, way too early— like the middle of the night. Buried in the subconscious is that concern for an approaching deadline or an unresolved family issue. Like a running car engine, these worries are propelling our adrenals to pump out cortisol, and our mind takes off at 3 AM. How do we let go of such concerns?

During the various stages of sleep, the mind processes and orders the events of the day, connections and memories are strengthened or eliminated, waste products are removed from the brain, the body's cells and tissues are repaired, and hormones are released that regulate our appetite. It's no surprise that even one night without these essential functions can have major ramifications the next day.

Relaxation and stress reduction make up Step Two of the Sleep Away the Pounds Program. This step is all about reducing stress and calming your mind so you can get a good night's sleep—each and every night. We also want you to learn how to reduce the stress hormones that pack on the pounds, especially on the belly. The tools in this chapter can help you effectively deal with the mental or emotional issues that stress you out or keep you awake. Exercises follow that can help you change your responses to life's stresses and let go of your cares and concerns to achieve balance in mind, body, and spirit.

HOLISTICALLY SPEAKING: STRESS AND IMMUNITY

Stress is the mental, emotional, or physical strain caused, for example, by anxiety, emotional issues, or overwork. Excess stress in our lives does more damage than just a poor night of sleep. Besides the weight gain that can result from too much stress and too little sleep, your immune system will also pay a price. As whole beings, we cannot separate ourselves into parts that are separate. As much as we like to categorize parts of ourselves—for example, our digestive system and circulatory system, our mind versus our body—these separations are really just artificial constructs. What happens in our digestive system affects our circulatory system, just as what happens in our mind affects our body. Ask yourself—where does your mind end and your body begin?

When we are stressed, our bodies release the hormone cortisol.

We were given this mechanism for times when stress meant we were being stalked by a mountain lion or starving to death. And while some people still experience life-and-death stress on a daily basis, most of us experience stress that is not life-threatening. Though these non-life-threatening stresses may be related to work, relationships, or traffic, our body still reacts as if we are being hunted by the mountain lion. Our fight-or-flight response kicks in, and our bodies are flooded with cortisol to help us flee the scene or attack back when that mountain lion strikes.

If we are constantly stressed, then our levels of cortisol stay elevated. Cortisol, while useful in short-term, life-threatening situations, has many negative health effects when it's constantly released into the bloodstream. A powerful immunosuppressant, cortisol breaks down lymphoid tissue, reducing the number of T-helper cells and natural killer cells, which are immune cells. It also inhibits the amount of interferon, a naturally occurring antiviral agent. Have you ever had a stressful event that you powered through, only to find that you fell ill as soon as it was over? This type of experience is consistent with the results of one study in students, which found that those who experienced the most serious illness were also those who experienced the most stress, both academically and socially.

LIFE BALANCE QUIZ

Just how balanced is your life? Take the Life Balance Quiz to determine just where you may need to put in some work to live a healthier, more balanced life.

Answer true or false to the following questions:

1. I have more than enough time to do what I want to do.
2. I am on a health regimen that helps me feel energized.
3. I look forward to every day.
4. There are no people in my life (at home or at work) who drain me.

5. I love my home (location, contents, the feel, the style).
6. I have no clutter in my home and/or office.
7. I have a life pursuing what I want to do instead of what I should do.
8. My work is satisfying and rewarding.
9. I take at least two weeklong vacations a year.
10. I do not work on weekends.
11. I get plenty of sleep.
12. I have plenty of quality time with my children and/or the people who matter to me.
13. I have at least one hobby or pastime outside of my work and family activities.
14. I eat foods that make me feel energized instead of sluggish.
15. I have the space to take at least fifteen minutes of silence a day.
16. I have friends who are easy to be with and a joy to spend time with.
17. I carry no heavy emotional burdens or addictive behaviors.

Give yourself one point for every time you said true. If you answered true more often than false (a score of at least 9), you are probably living a well-balanced life. If you scored 8 or less, your lifestyle may need some fine-tuning.

In that case, start by letting yourself off the hook. With the pace of our lives today, many of us would flunk this quiz. The important thing to focus on is what to do about it. The first step is to take two days off immediately to relax and regroup. That may be hard, but it's crucial. During your time off, ask yourself, *What am I hating, tolerating, or resenting about the current state of my life?* Make a list and generate ideas about how to start correcting these aspects of your life. That is the first step. The second is to implement those changes and begin to rebalance your life.

Stress, insomnia, and the accompanying health effects are often the result of an imbalance in our lives. When we integrate all aspects of our selves, we take a more holistic approach to life. The journey starts with our physical body and health, and includes proper nutrition, exercise, and rest. For many people, this is the most difficult change to make, but the results are easy to see. It is a bit more challenging to change the parts of us we can't see. Our emotional health is complex and often hard to access. Initial work may involve a therapist. Daily support for our emotional health includes those things we already know make us feel good—time for our families and loved ones, time for ourselves and the things we enjoy doing.

STRESSFUL EVENTS: HOW THEY RANK

Drs. Thomas H. Holmes and Richard H. Rahe, psychiatrists at the University of Washington Medical School, have devised a scale of measurement for stressful events. These various events are rated numerically on the right so you can add up your score. A total of 200 or more units in one year is considered to be predictive of the likeliness of developing a serious disease.

Death of spouse	100
Divorce	73
Marital separation	65
Jail term	63
Death of close family member	63
Personal injury or illness	53
Marriage	50
Fired at work	47
Marital reconciliation	45
Retirement	45
Change in health of family member	44

Pregnancy	40
Sexual difficulties	39
Gain of new family	39
Business adjustment	39
Change in financial state	38
Death of close friend	37
Change to different line of work	36
Increased number of arguments with spouse	35
Large mortgage	31
Foreclosure of mortgage or loan	30
Change in responsibilities at work	29
Son or daughter leaving home	29
Trouble with in-laws	29
Outstanding personal achievement	28
Spouse begins or stops work	26
Begin or end school	26
Change in living conditions	25
Revision of personal habits	24
Trouble with boss	23
Change in work hours or conditions	20
Change in residence	20
Change in schools	20
Change in recreation	19
Change in church activities	19
Change in social activities	18
Small mortgage	17
Change in sleeping habits	16
Change in number of family get-togethers	15
Change in eating habits	15
Vacation	13
Christmas	12
Minor violations of the law	11

Mental health can involve challenging work and careers, but it doesn't end there. It is important to remember that there is always more to learn. Take a class, learn a new skill, read a historical book, attend a lecture. Like our muscles, the mind must be used to stay strong and vibrant. Our spirituality is the deepest part of us and involves our soul. For some, religion is a way to practice spirituality. Other people have their own ways of accessing their souls and rejoicing in the world around them. Whatever the method, our spirituality gives us meaning and purpose and involves relinquishing some control over our lives. This sense of just letting go of control reduces stress and allows us to experience a greater sense of tranquillity.

EMOTIONS AND SLEEP: ANXIETY MANAGEMENT

In our hectic 24/7 world, stress is the main culprit for those sleepless nights. And the more stress you have, the more worn down and stressed out you become! A vicious cycle is born—high stress leads to trouble sleeping, which elevates your stress levels and makes you less able to deal with anxiety.

Psychological stressors, such as upcoming events of importance, job or school deadlines, or relationship issues, may interfere with sleep. As soon as we hit the pillow, all of the day's worries start swirling around in our minds. Often this is because bedtime is the only time of the day that we're truly still and receptive to our thoughts. Or we may fall asleep but wake up early with our minds hard at work and possibly not even on the stressful situation. We may be unaware of the worry or concern buried in the subconscious. Therefore, it is important to break the connection between the day, with all its stressors, and nighttime, before hitting the sheets.

So what do you do to jump ship and move to calmer seas?

OVERCOMING ANXIETY AND AN OVERACTIVE MIND

A chattering mind or fear of not being able to sleep can keep you awake half the night. Easing into sleep and staying asleep can sometimes seem impossible because the harder we try, the harder it is to go to sleep. The following tips may help you overcome two common sleep problems.

• To calm a chattering mind, slowly repeat a relaxing word or phrase. You could choose something like "soooo sleepy," or "deep sleep," or "I'm getting sleepier, and sleepier, and sleepier." Or you might sing yourself a favorite lullaby, either in your mind or out loud. These techniques give the left hemisphere of your brain what it likes—repetitive words and phrases that get the brain into slow-wave mode that takes you into sleep.

• To overcome sleep anxiety, learn to think new thoughts about going to sleep. Psychophysiological insomnia is the result of anxiety that comes from a few nights of insomnia. This can set you up to fear another sleepless night. Then, if you awaken for any reason, your body may start pumping out stress hormones such as cortisol and adrenaline that can keep you awake for hours. If you find yourself thinking, "I've got to get to sleep or I'll be a wreck tomorrow," you can replace such a thought with, "When I'm ready, I'll get to sleep. After all, I don't have to have this night's sleep." It's important to take the pressure off getting to sleep right away. It's best to shift your attention from *making* yourself get to sleep to *allowing* yourself to go to sleep. This helps the brain slow down so you can relax and drift off to sleep naturally.

Luckily, several effective behavioral strategies exist for managing and letting go of your worries. In addition to the relaxation methods mentioned in this chapter, anxiety management may be accomplished by writing or journaling. A simple list of the stressors of the day, along with a brief plan to deal with them, may be just what you need to put the day, and yourself, to rest.

THE STRESS-MANAGEMENT TRILOGY

So now that you know how detrimental stress is, what do you do about it? Stress isn't just a mental issue; therefore, stress management must center on the physical, psychological, and spiritual aspects to truly be effective. All of the methods highlighted in this chapter focus on aspects of the physical, psychological, and spiritual, with many techniques emphasizing one area more strongly. When deciding what approach works best for you, you may want to combine aspects of different techniques, giving equal attention to all aspects of your being to assure that you are taking a whole-person approach to stress management, thus covering all your bases.

Caring for the physical, psychological, and spiritual aspects of our selves allows us to manage stress in a holistic manner. By balancing the attention and energy we give to each aspect of our being, we can use all parts of our being to counteract stress and bring peace and health into our lives.

THE PHYSICAL SIDE OF
STRESS MANAGEMENT

The physical part of stress management is one that most of us are familiar with. In order to be healthy mentally, emotionally, and spiritually, we must maintain physical health. Remember, it's all one and the same! Eating right, getting regular exercise, taking nutritional supplements as needed, and getting restful sleep will elevate our mood, enhance our immune function, and allow us to accomplish our goals (weight-related and beyond) and enjoy our lives. Being sick is a huge source of stress, because when we're ill, everything we want and need to do gets pushed down to the bottom of the list. The old adage *Health is wealth* is the absolute truth. Because the bulk of the Sleep Away the Pounds Program is dedicated to strategies for relaxation, restful sleep, and weight loss, this chapter is devoted especially to psychological and spiritual aspects of ourselves that we so often neglect.

DEEP-BREATHING EXERCISE

1. Lie on the floor in a comfortable position. Bend your knees and move your feet about ten inches apart, with your toes turned slightly outward. Keep your spine straight and the small of your back flat on the floor.
2. Place one hand on your abdomen and one hand on your chest.
3. Inhale slowly and deeply through your nose, filling your abdomen with air and pushing up your hands as much as is comfortable. Your chest should move only a little and only with your abdomen.
4. Exhale through your mouth, making a soft whooshing sound like the wind blowing gently.
5. Continue this process of deep breathing for five to ten minutes at a time, once or twice a day.
6. At the end of your deep breathing, compare how you felt before you started with how you feel now.

THE PSYCHOLOGICAL SIDE OF
STRESS MANAGEMENT

Psychological or mental vitality is essential for maintaining a positive outlook on life and minimizing stress and anxiety. Here are some suggestions for psychological health.

Avoid too many changes at one time. Order your life in a way that you do not experience too much change all at once. For example, if you are going through a divorce and have just moved to a new home, now is probably not a good time to change jobs (see Stressful Events: How They Rank on page 48). Put off new changes until you've adapted to the current changes in your life.

Recognize your personal stress signals, such as a racing heart, clenched jaw, grinding teeth, tensed muscles, awakening in the night with a racing mind, or nail biting. When you notice these signals, take time to counteract your stress response by doing relaxation exercises, such as meditating, deep breathing, and systematic tensing and relaxation of the muscles. These exercises can be effective for managing your stress even if there is only time to practice them briefly.

Watch what you allow your mind to dwell on. If your mind continuously plays a negative record of events or words, it will affect your ability to sleep as well as your overall health. Learn to interrupt your negative thoughts and insert a positive, health-supporting mental dialogue instead. Think about it—if you cannot tell where the mind ends and the body begins, then where do the negative thoughts that originate in your mind come to a stop? (To calm your mind, you could also try the Bach Flower Essence white chestnut, which is used to calm a chattering mind. Put several drops under your tongue as needed. It can be found at most health food stores.)

Relaxation Techniques

Relaxation techniques include some of the oldest insomnia remedies we know. Simple relaxation involves prayer, meditation (see page 57), a hot bath, soothing music, a good book, or exercises such as Progressive Muscle Relaxation or Brain Entrainment. Meditation has been proven to have a profound effect on the body, mind, and spirit. While deep in meditation, heart and respiration rates slow, brain waves are smoother and less sporadic, and many people report feeling a profound sense of calm and well-being. Though it's common to use television to unwind, TV viewing is not considered an effective relaxation technique, as it tends to stimulate the brain. Since when did the evening news or an action-packed show make you feel relaxed?

PROGRESSIVE MUSCLE RELAXATION TECHNIQUE

1. Sit in a chair with as little strain on your lower back and abdomen as possible. Place your feet comfortably on the floor, about one foot apart. Lift your hands and drop them to your thighs. Allow your head to move slowly to a comfortable position. Close your eyes.

2. Take a deep breath and gently exhale. Allow your breath to be one with your body.

3. Continue breathing in this manner and slightly tense your hands, arms, and shoulders. Concentrate on how this feels. Then relax your shoulders, arms, and forearms. Relax your wrists, hands, and fingers next; imagine a feeling of relaxation flowing through your entire body to your toes.

4. Contract and tense your scalp, forehead, eyelids, jaw muscles and the areas around your eyes and mouth. Now

imagine a peaceful, calm feeling flowing through your neck, shoulders, arms, hands, and on into your chest, abdomen, and down through your hips, legs, calves, feet, and toes.

5. Take a deep breath and tighten the muscles in your chest and abdomen. Then exhale and allow your chest and abdomen to completely relax. Imagine relaxing internally, through your organs, glands, and cells. Next, tighten your hips, legs, feet, and toes. Then slowly release the tension through your hips, legs, feet, and toes.

6. Imagine your toes to be like faucets. See yourself turning the faucets on and letting all remaining tension drain from your body out your toes. As it washes away, imagine a deep sense of relaxation flowing from your scalp down through your forehead, eyelids, face, and jaw muscles. Picture it flowing down through your neck, shoulders, arms, and hands. Allow this feeling to continue through your chest and abdomen, hips, legs, and on to your toes. See yourself as completely relaxed.

7. Imagine that you are at complete peace with yourself and the world around you.

8. Now open your eyes slowly. Stretch your arms above your head and take a deep breath. Exhale and let your arms drop.

Brain Entrainment: Sound, Music, and the Brain

For many years, French ear, nose, and throat specialist Dr. Alfred Tomatis has been studying the ways the brain processes incoming sounds. One of his studies involved a Benedictine monastery where a new abbot eliminated the monks' traditional six to eight hours of daily chanting. Without the chants, Dr. Tomatis observed, the monks suddenly became listless and fatigued. To find out why, he studied

the sounds of the chanting and found that the high-frequency over-
tones actually provided electroneural stimulation to the brain. So, he
concluded, because the sounds of these Gregorian chants appeared
to naturally recharge the monks' bodies and brains, their elimination
resulted in an enormous decline of energy. (Remember when *Chant:
The Benedictine Monks of Santo Domingo de Silos* topped the music charts
in the early 1990s? Perhaps the positive brain stimulation received

BASIC MEDITATION

Follow these steps for ten to twenty minutes twice a day for a
calmer mind and a better night's sleep:

1. Find a quiet place where you won't be disturbed.
2. Choose a word or short phrase that is firmly rooted in
   your belief system; for example, a Christian person can
   use the name of Jesus or a phrase such as *Lord have
   mercy*, a Jewish person can use the name of God or a
   phrase from the Torah, a nonreligious person can use a
   word such as *one, peace,* or *love.*
3. Sit quietly in a comfortable position.
4. Close your eyes.
5. Relax your muscles. Lower your shoulders and gently
   roll your head a couple of times.
6. Breathe slowly and naturally and repeat the first part of
   your focus word or phrase as you inhale and the last part
   of your focus word as you exhale.
7. Assume a passive attitude. Don't worry about how
   you're doing. When other thoughts come to your mind,
   as they inevitably will, let them go and return to your
   focus word.
8. Continue for ten to twenty minutes.

when listening to this music was what attracted so many people.) Evidence from additional studies suggests that various types of music have a restorative effect on the brain and body. Beside Gregorian chants, effective music includes classical, baroque, certain types of jazz, and relaxing instrumental music.

The next time you're looking for a way to recharge, pop in a CD of this type of music, find a cozy spot, and let the music fill your body and soul.

THE SPIRITUAL SIDE OF STRESS MANAGEMENT

Historically, stress has been lowered by religious and spiritual practices. This effect may be due to the fact that spiritual beliefs foster many stress-reducing beliefs and attitudes such as optimism, appreciation, commitment, trust, empathy, forgiveness, and altruism. Religious and spiritual beliefs also provide meaning and purpose, placing stressful situations in perspective and producing calming effects. Dr. Herbert Benson of Harvard Medical School believes that the tendency for humans to engage in religious beliefs and prayer is encoded in our physiology.

Spirituality means different things to different people. For some, it means being part of an organized religion and taking part in services, traditions, and activities that are components of the religious worship. For others, spirituality takes shape in prayer, singing sacred music, scripture reading, meditating, visiting nature, and other forms of personal reflection and interaction with God or a Higher Power. Many people practice both religion and personal forms of spirituality. The objective is to have some way in which you get in touch with your spirit and God or your Higher Power, which is the true purpose behind practicing any form of spirituality.

Prayer and Closing the Day

During our fast-paced days, we experience thousands of interactions, communications, and observations. Whether conscious of these experiences or not, we are processing all this information in our mind. The result of all this "uploading" can be fatigue, anxiety, and an inability to relax and sleep well, especially if that day contained any especially stressful interactions. It's no wonder that when we shut our eyes at night, it's hard to turn off our mind.

In order to close out the day, it's important to "download" some of what we took in. Exercises such as meditation, deep breathing, stretching, and relaxation techniques are very helpful. But one of the most relaxing and rejuvenating techniques is prayer. For some people, prayers are recited or read from a prayer book; for others it's simply conversation with God or their Higher Source. Prayers may be well known such as the Lord's Prayer, or spontaneous words of praise, adoration, thankfulness, or they can be requests for a specific need. They can be long and imploring or short and to the point. For example, our friend Lou Ann King, executive director of Optimum Health Institute in Austin, Texas, says sometimes her prayers are very short; they go something like this: "Please, God"; or, "Help me"; or, "Bless them." Prayers may also be scripture, hymns, or poems expressed as a meditation. The function of prayer is to let go of your cares and issues, and to reconnect with your spiritual self and with the Source of Love.

As explained by Saint Theophan, "All of your inner disorder is due to the dislocation of your powers, the mind and the heart each going their own way. You must unite the mind with the heart; then the tumult of your thoughts will cease, and you will acquire a rudder to guide the ship of your soul, a lever with which to put all your inner world in movement." To ensure a healthy sleep routine, it's important to consciously bring the day to an end. After all the evening's work and routine are done—or maybe not finished but left for later because it's time for bed—find a comfortable place to relax. Take a moment to review the day without judgment; simply focus on the events. You may wish to play some relaxing music as you reflect. You may also want to engage in breathing exercises or gentle stretching. For the final closing of your day, a prayer that includes an unloading of your cares and concerns, and perhaps a poem or song, can help you to release unresolved issues and find a place of inner peace.

SOME PRAYERS TO END THE DAY

Following are examples of two Celtic prayers from *The Edge of Glory: Prayers in the Celtic Tradition* by David Adam and a poem you could use at the close of your day:

First Prayer

Spirit be about my head
Spirit peace around me shed
Spirit light about my way
Spirit guardian night and day
Come Holy Dove
Cover with Love

Second Prayer

I weave a silence onto my lips
I weave a silence into my mind
I weave a silence within my heart
I close my ears to distractions
I close my eyes to attractions
I close my heart to temptations
Calm me O Lord as you stilled the storm
Still me O Lord, keep me from harm
Let all the tumult within me cease
Enfold me Lord in your peace

A Poem (from "The Brewing of Soma" by John Greenleaf Whittier)

> Drop thy still dews of quietness,
>   Till all our strivings cease;
> Take from our souls the strain and stress,
> And let our ordered lives confess
>   The beauty of Thy peace.
>
> Breathe through the heats of our desire
>   Thy coolness and Thy balm;
> Let sense be dumb, let flesh retire;
> Speak through the earthquake, wind, and fire,
>   O still, small voice of calm!

Forgiveness: A Powerful Healing Practice

One of the fundamental themes in religious teachings worldwide is the power of forgiveness. The process of forgiving others and yourself for mistakes and wrongdoings is one of the most crucial steps in unburdening your mind and lightening your load. Walking around with anger and frustration bottled up inside is not healthy or helpful. If you can replace blame and hurt with forgiveness and love, your physical and mental health will benefit immensely.

The Aramaic definition of *forgiveness* is "letting go of my demands that I may unconditionally love this person." In other words, you accept others with their faults. Though our relationships have a deep effect on our well-being, it is important to remember that our relationships are not the source of our well-being. Given that understanding, any time we demonstrate anything contrary to love, it hurts us spiritually, physically, and emotionally. And though we cannot control how other people treat us, it is up to us how we define our experiences. By finding ways to let go, we can learn to forgive and replace negativity with love, unloading negative emotions and replacing them with internal peace.

If someone has disappointed or hurt you, act upon the principle of forgiveness. It's not just for the other person that you forgive; in fact, it may not be for that person at all that you make this choice. Anger, bitterness, or resentment can eat at your soul and do far more damage than just hindering a good night's sleep. Forgiveness frees us from our past and present hurts. And it's vital for our physical and emotional health.

In order to keep his brothers from experiencing worrying dreams, Saint Benedict recommended "they make peace before sunset if they had quarreled." Indeed, we all know how difficult good sleep can be if we have an intense discussion or argument with someone that remains unresolved at bedtime. It is important to reconcile these differences before going to bed, and put off all unsettled discussions until the following day. This does not mean that the conflict is necessarily resolved, only that a kind of truce has been called and you are consciously letting go of the issues at hand for the night. This does not need to involve the other person you are in conflict with. An open mind and heart, a moment dedicated to letting go, and a prayer of your own choosing or creation are all that are required.

The objective is to let go of our demands and expectations of other people. To accomplish this, it's important to keep our focus on the true source of life, which is love. Bitterness and resentment keep us trapped and stop our ability to resolve relational issues, grow, and become who we were meant to be.

Remember, you always have a choice to move from a reactive/responsive orientation to a creative/active lifestyle. Moving to a creative orientation transcends the past and allows you to grow in your present situation.

TURNED OFF TO SPIRITUAL MATTERS?

Some people have had negative religious experiences in their past that have turned them off to the whole topic of spirituality. Another reason people may have trouble embracing spirituality today may be that it cannot be explained in scientific terms. According to science, reality is only that which can be explained with the senses—sight, sound, taste, smell, and touch. Since spirituality is not something that most of us experience through these sensations, it becomes difficult for us to take seriously. Therefore, we may not have learned to relate to life on a spiritual dimension.

We must ask what price we pay for ignoring our spiritual needs. We can look for our own ways to cope with stress and pain. But many times the external events, situations, substances, or things we choose as coping methods end up being addictive. At the point where we find a compulsive habitual desire forming for anything, then we have to admit that the way we have chosen to meet our needs or cope with life's frustrations isn't working. If stress is threatening to sink our ship, and nights of endless tossing and turning in bed seem to have no answer, perhaps it is time to look beyond our familiar methods of coping. Actually, this can be seen as an opportunity to examine the whole issue of spirituality and to experience personal spirituality in a way that is life-giving and able to take us to new peace and meaning.

REFRAMING: CREATING POSITIVE INTENTIONS

Our behaviors are purposeful. Despite our feelings that life is happening to us, quite the opposite is true—we are happening to the world around us. All of us engage in some behaviors that we know are not very effective. Many times, we would like to change these behaviors, but that change seems difficult.

Behaviors, whether internal or external, were learned because that was the best way we knew how to deal with a situation at the time it arose. Many behaviors are learned in childhood, when tools for dealing with these situations are limited. Even after we grow up and understand better strategies for handling issues, those old behaviors often stick around. Unless we identify the purpose for our actions or reactions—also known as behaviors—and find alternatives that make sense, we will continue to do what we have always done. Since these behaviors are habitual, it doesn't work to try to change the behavior without first exploring its purpose, and then working on both the behavior and its intention. A process called reframing can help us create new, more effective behaviors from old habits.

Tim, for example, practiced the reframing process after identifying a dietary behavior he wanted to change. He had an enormous sweet tooth, often eating two or three desserts a day. Not only was his waistline paying for it, but he often felt tired and mentally sluggish from the rapid rise and fall of his blood sugar after eating sweets. Tim learned about reframing, and practiced the following steps to create better eating habits.

Step 1: Identify the behavior, attitude, or symptom you want to change. The behavior Tim wanted to change was his over-consumption of sweets.

Step 2: Ask yourself the reason or intention for your behavior, attitude, or symptom. In asking himself why he reached for desserts all day, Tim realized that these foods made him feel happy and gave him a sense of comfort, while satisfying cravings for sugar.

Step 3: Come up with three or more new ways to satisfy your intentions effectively. Tim's ideas included eating fruit when he was craving sweets, eating small snacks throughout the day to balance his blood sugar, allowing himself a limit of three desserts per week (instead of per day!) so he would not feel completely deprived, and making a list of nonfood sources of comfort. His list included a cup of tea and a good book, a leisurely walk around the neighborhood, e-mailing a friend, gardening, and deep-breathing exercises.

Step 4: Make a commitment to begin the new behaviors now. Because Tim was tired of feeling tired and wanted to shed some pounds, he was committed to beginning the reframing process immediately. He realized that it took a firm commitment to start right away, knowing that the longer he continued with the old habits, the harder it would be to change.

Step 5: Don't rush to begin all the changes at once. Start practicing one of the new behaviors today, then add the second behavior, and incorporate the third change as appropriate. Trying to change everything at once would be overwhelming and might cause you to revert to your old habits. To begin his process, Tim went to the store and loaded up on fruit. For the next few days, he replaced one dessert each day with a piece of fruit. Then he began replacing an additional dessert each day with an activity from his comfort list. Throughout this time, Tim also tried to eat more frequently throughout the day, so as to maintain his blood sugar and prevent cravings. After a couple of weeks, Tim began limiting his dessert intake to three sweets a week. It wasn't easy, and occasionally he slipped, but Tim stayed committed, and he succeeded in turning unwanted habits into effective new behaviors.

LIVING ON PURPOSE

Why are you here? This is surely not the first time you have asked yourself that question. It is a fundamental struggle for people everywhere. We all wonder why we are alive and what our purpose is on earth. Some people seem to be born knowing what they should do with their lives; others come to it down a longer, harder path. What is important is that you spend time doing self-exploration and figuring out what your purpose is. If you feel like you are just going through the motions, doing things you have to do instead of things you want to do, then you are living off purpose. Those who are living on purpose, on the other hand, feel a sense of meaning and are better able to deal with change. They experience a sense of fulfillment, reward, and vitality, and their performance and satisfaction in what they do are strong. When people feel that they are living in a way that is consistent with their purpose, they are less likely to grab quick fixes that will provide short-term fulfillment, such as an alcoholic drink or fattening food.

Unfortunately, a chapter in a book can't tell you your purpose in life. That takes self-reflection, listening, brainstorming, prayer, and sometimes trial and error. For those of us who aren't born with a conscious knowledge of our purpose, practicing the introspection or inner work that will give us this understanding is one of the most important things we can do with our lives. After all, once we are aware of our purpose, it will provide guidance for everything else we do. To facilitate this process of understanding, focus on the following areas, and reflect upon how much enjoyment and achievement you feel in each. Any answer other than "a lot" indicates that this is an area of your life that may need some evaluation and adjustment in order to get you back on purpose:

- Work
- Relationships with family and friends

- Relationship with significant other
- Physical health
- Emotional health
- Intellectual growth
- Spiritual growth

UNDERSTANDING THE SOURCE
OF STRESS AND LETTING GO

It is all too easy to put the onus of our stress and anxiety onto the people and world around us: "I'm stressed out because my boss made me work late," or "I'm having a bad day because my spouse didn't help with the housework this morning," or even "I can't take one more day of this traffic!" But ask yourself: Is it the events in your life that are the cause of your tension, or is it the emotional response you have to those stimuli?

Lester Levenson, creator of the Sedona Method, decided to try some self-examination after suffering a massive heart attack. During this period, he came to realize that his own responses to the events in the world around him were the major cause of his stress and subsequent health issues. The Sedona Method is a process by which emotional responses to external stimuli are identified, processed, and released. When we let go of the negative emotion, the stress and anxiety that follow it are also relinquished.

Studies at the Laboratory of Cognitive Psychobiology of the State University of New York, and the Department of Psychology and Social Relations at Harvard University, have concluded that the Sedona Method is a highly effective antidote to stress. Three and a half months after the initial research, a follow-up study showed that the participants were still experiencing dramatic reductions in stress.

GETTING DOWN TO THE ROOT OF STRESS: OUR SYNOPSIS OF THE SEDONA METHOD

Step One: Focus. Select an area in your life that has a large emotional component for you. It may be your job, family, an illness, a recent loss ... whatever feels very emotionally charged.

Step Two: Feel. Ask yourself, *What am I feeling right now?* Most feelings actually fit into a few main categories.

There are six categories, or root feelings, that Levenson identifies as being the most toxic. Note the feeling(s) that you experience:

- Anger. Other emotions associated with anger are aggression, annoyance, argumentativeness, defiance, disgust, frustration, hatefulness, impatience, jealousy, outrage, resentment, spitefulness, stubbornness, vengefulness, viciousness, and violence.

- Apathy. This can include boredom, carelessness, defeatism, depression, discouragement, disillusionment, futility, hopelessness, powerlessness, resignation, and worthlessness.

- Fear. This can include anxiety, apprehensiveness, doubtfulness, inhibition, insecurity, nervousness, panic, shakiness, worry, and feeling trapped.

- Grief. This can include feelings of abandonment, abuse, guilt, anguish, shame, betrayal, embarrassment, helplessness, hurt, isolation, neglect, rejection, and sadness.

- Lust. The main feeling behind lust is *I want*. Accompanying emotions are anticipation, craving, demanding, desire, feeling devious, feeling driven, envy, frustration, greed, manipulation, obsession, ruthlessness, selfishness, and wickedness.

- Pride. Pride can cause you to act aloof, arrogant, boastful, clever, contemptuous, cool, critical, judgmental, righteous, rigid, self-satisfied, snobbish, spoiled, superior, selfish, unforgiving, and vain.

While you focus on your feelings and their root causes, check in with your body and look for physical responses. A rapid heartbeat, tension, perspiration, tears, nausea, and other strong bodily reactions will testify to the deep effect that the particular emotion has on your entire being.

Step Three: Feel your feeling. Before you are able to release a feeling, you must feel it. Instead of stuffing the feeling back, allow it to surface, and accept any physical response you might have, such as crying, feeling sad, or becoming angry.

Step Four: Could you let go? As you are experiencing this feeling, ask yourself, *Could I let this feeling go?* Recognize that emotions are not who we are. Your true self is separate from your emotions. One of the ways you know this is that you are able to feel the feeling at the same time you are asking yourself to let it go. Once you understand that the emotion is not intrinsically a part of you, you can see the possibility of releasing that feeling.

Step Five: Would you? After realizing that it is possible to release an emotion, you must assess if you are willing to let it go. Honesty is important here, as you may be too angry or upset to let go of the emotion. Even if you answer no, continue with the process. Eventually, you will become tired of this emotion and its negative effects, and you will truly be willing to let it go.

Step Six: When? Once you realize it is possible to let go of the feeling, ask yourself, *When will I be ready to let it go?* Can you let it go in a few minutes . . . in a week? After thinking about this for a bit, just let the answer come.

Step Seven: Release. The final step in this process is to release the feeling. When your answer is finally yes, the feeling will go. This should feel like a huge relief. Accompanying it may be laughter or tears or the feeling that a burden has been lifted. You may also notice that you are sleeping better. In addition, other emotions may surface as you release this one. If so, just go through the same process with those other feelings in order to release them as well.

Though this method may be challenging at first, the more you practice, the more effective you will become at using these tools. The result is that you will have a healthy and therapeutic way to deal with your emotions and eliminate the stress, anxiety, and health issues that piggyback onto your negative emotions.

The Sedona Method is based on the premise that people have three ways in which they deal with a feeling: They *suppress it*, they *express it*, or they try to *escape it*. All three of these methods have negative consequences. *Suppressing* a feeling permits it to fester within us, and creates an internal environment of tension, anxiety, and depression. *Expressing*, or venting, a feeling is often thought of as the best way to deal with it. But expressing an emotion does not make it go away. In fact, if we express ourselves by blowing up, we often feel guilty afterward, leaving us with yet another negative emotion to contend with. Many of us thus turn to *escape* to handle our feelings; calling a friend, watching television, eating, drinking, or using drugs are all ways to divert our attention away from our real feelings. But like suppression and expression, escaping a feeling does not make it go away.

According to Levenson and numerous research studies, the healthiest way to handle our emotions is to *release* them. If you are able to understand the emotion and let it go, it is no longer lingering and causing damage. This is the principle of the Sedona Method, as described in the box below. By practicing this method over time, you will find that you are calmer and more productive. The cumulative effect of this practice is to reach a state of imperturbability wherein people, experiences, and emotions are no longer able to throw you off balance. The Sedona Method offers a set of tools for dealing with stimuli in such a way that you are able to remain clearheaded, discharge negative feelings, and stay emotionally centered.

THE HEART OF THE MATTER

When our body, mind, and soul come into harmony, our sleep patterns also become smoother and more restorative. By getting out of our heads, we are able to get into our hearts. A heart researcher, Dr. J. Andrew Armour, has been studying the way the heart affects the rest of the body and mind. Armour discovered that the heart has its own nervous system, which functions like a tiny brain. This network of neurons, neurotransmitters, proteins, and support cells enables the heart to operate and process information independently of the cranial brain or nervous system. In fact, as long as they are supplied with oxygen, heart cells will continue to beat after being removed from the body. The heart sends its own signals to the brain, which help regulate the nervous system, organ function, and cognitive processes. In other words, the brain is not the only organ controlling and directing the body. The heart isn't just taking orders, but also helping run the show. In the heart is life.

The Institute of HeartMath is a research and educational organization that has developed simple tools to relieve stress. The basic idea behind these exercises is that by using our heart to deal with the situations in our lives, called "heart intelligence," we can bring our mind and body into balance. The physiological premise of this belief stems from studies on heart rate variability and emotion. Because of the way that emotions affect our nervous system, and therefore our heart, heart rate variability can show a direct physical response to an emotion. In these studies, participants are hooked up to heart rate monitors, and different emotions are elicited. When a stressful emotion is evoked, the participant's heart rate has an irregular, jagged, incoherent pattern. When the participant shifts to a more positive emotional state, the heart rhythm pattern changes to a smoother, wavelike, coherent pattern.

This understanding of emotions, stress, and heart rate can assist us in becoming more whole and balanced. As you can imagine, a jagged, incoherent heart rate does not lend itself to a good night's sleep.

Living from Your Heart

What does it mean to you to "live from the heart"? Imagine if your ideas, emotions, choices, and responses were generated from your heart instead of your mind. How might that affect your ability to appreciate the people and experiences you encounter? Going from the head to the heart stops the chattering in the mind, and enables us to see ourself and our life with greater clarity.

Living from the heart is a unique notion and different for each individual. A common thread is the intention to embrace life with sincerity and appreciation. When you are feeling appreciative of the world around you, and the people you interact with, it is almost impossible to feel stressed about those same people and experiences. When you let someone know how appreciative you feel, you are spreading love and positive energy. Sincerity is essential because it motivates us and helps turn our desires into actions. If you approach each day with a sense of sincerity about your intentions, you will find the power to bring coherence into your life—aligning your heart and mind in a way that enables you to focus on your purpose.

Remember that like attracts like. If you live your life with positive intent, and use your heart to guide you, you will attract loving, positive people and situations into your life. We tend to surround

APPRECIATION FROM THE HEART

Consider a challenging situation in your life. It can be a current issue you are dealing with, something you dealt with in the past, or even a situation you expect to be challenging in the future.

1. Describe the challenging situation in words, writing it down on paper.

2. Write down three things that you can appreciate about this situation.

3. Write down up to three things about this situation that you would consider draining or negative.

4. Carefully read over your deficit list. Are there any deficits that can be transformed into assets? Are there any deficits that can be neutralized with a different perspective?

5. Go through these steps and pick out the challenging issue. You will be surprised at how much good you can find in a situation that may seem hopeless.

Remember that appreciation is an easy emotion to feel. Rarely do we have the kind of emotional walls built against it that we do with more harmful emotions. No matter how bleak the situation may feel, try to find at least one thing you can appreciate about it. Your mind will remember your appreciation of a situation more easily than a negative emotion, because the heart and mind are willing and able to go there.

ourselves with people of the same ilk. Just as negativity becomes self-perpetuating, so do happiness and peace. When you practice living from the heart, you bring coherence into your own life.

So how do you live from the heart? One of the key elements is to practice stepping outside your normal way of seeing things. Most of us live in our heads, and react to the world around us in a predictable way. That is, we respond to events and people habitually, in the way we have always responded. Some of us analyze our lives and relationships constantly; others just take it all in, without much dissection. Either way, it is helpful to step back at times and take stock of your life and how you are living it. See the box on page 73 to practice living with appreciation and using your heart to guide you.

CHOICES

As you learn more about the links among sleep, stress, and obesity, you may be thinking about making a few changes—to your diet, your sleep patterns, and your lifestyle. Change itself, even if it's change for the better, is a source of stress. When we make changes in our lives, it is always easier to fall back to the patterns we are familiar and comfortable with than to forge ahead into the unknown. This is the difference between what is called the choice response and the default response.

An example of these different responses can be seen in the story of Sarah's struggle to lose weight. Sarah had been battling extra pounds for years, and as part of a New Year's resolution to finally lose weight, she had gone to see a nutritionist. The nutritionist helped Sarah to develop an eating plan and exercise routine that would allow her to achieve her weight loss goals. Armed with these tools and determined to shed some weight, Sarah began her new lifestyle. At first, it was easier than she thought. She enjoyed trying new foods and activities, and was fueled by the novelty of these changes. A few weeks into the weight loss plan, Sarah went to dinner with some friends. As she scanned the menu, she noticed some of her old favorites: fettuccine Alfredo, four-cheese macaroni, and prime rib with mashed potatoes. Sarah ordered the fettuccine Alfredo, which had been really good the last time she'd had it at this restaurant. When the drink orders went around the table, Sarah chimed in with a daiquiri. All the girls were doing it! Sarah ordered dessert and after-dinner drinks in a similar fashion—that is, with her default response. Instead of consciously thinking about the choices she was making, Sarah slipped back into her old patterns— her default. The next morning, she felt terrible about wrecking her new diet after such hard work over the previous weeks. But Sarah's friend talked her through it, explaining that people often slip up and relapse when they make new changes. It was up to Sarah to forge ahead with her commitment.

The next week, at a business lunch, Sarah was again faced with the decision of what to order at a restaurant filled with high-calorie foods she loved. This time, when she looked over the menu, she was thinking about her conversation with the nutritionist, and looking for foods that fit with her new diet plan. Choosing a salad, seared tuna, and an unsweetened iced tea, Sarah knew she was choosing a lunch that would be healthy and satisfying. She was making a choice response. Sarah was able to recognize that the choices she makes today affect the outcomes of tomorrow. These conscious and deliberate decisions will help her reach her goals.

People who practice choice responses are able to imagine how their present choices will affect their future. This ability to correlate present actions with the reality of your best possible future may take some practice (see page 76 for tips). All of us are creatures of habit, and it is always easier to rely on what we already know. But it is rewarding and often life changing to make the choice response.

CREATING A CHOICE RESPONSE

Using the example of dietary changes, here are some tips for moving away from a default response and toward a more conscious choice response.

Expectation. Get a plan early in mind about what you are going to do the next time you're tempted to eat foods you know aren't best for you. *Expect* that those temptations will arise.

Association. Correlate your actions with the outcome of your choices. In other words, recognize that what you eat today will affect your future health, either positively or negatively, depending on the food. Be as graphic as you can and try to actually feel what you would experience if you ate the thing you know you shouldn't eat—would it make you tired, sluggish, or spacey? Would it add excess calories, contributing to weight gain, or keep you awake half the night? If it's hard for you to think of negative physical sensations that may arise from eating this food, then imagine telling someone you hold yourself accountable to what you have eaten. Maybe it's your doctor, spouse, or friend—think about how you will feel when you tell them you have fallen off the wagon.

Visioning. Create positive associations for the foods that are good for you, and negative associations for the foods you want to avoid. A positive association may be: "Mineral water with a slice of lime is a refreshing drink that is better for me than alcohol, and it tastes great." A negative association might be: "The cheese-doozles are colored with orange dye and created in a lab . . . there are fifteen ingredients in them that I can't even pronounce and they'll make me fat." Make a collage or take pictures of yourself that represent a negative association and a positive one. Label them "my best self" and "my worst self." Choose which picture you want to create. The choices you make today will create your tomorrow.

Relapse and recovery. Change is hard, and an occasional slip is often inevitable. If you do slip, don't punish yourself. Recognize the mistake and resolve to do better next time. Get back up with a positive plan to make wise choices in the future by reviewing the steps above.

YOUR PERSONAL RELAXATION FORMULA

When you can't get to sleep because you're worried and feeling anxious, or depressed and feeling down, or confused and can't figure out what to do, you obviously aren't going to get to the root of your sleep trouble until you're able to work through the parts of your life that you're anxious or depressed about. There are numerous techniques for resolving stress, relaxing the mind, and enjoying restful sleep. The important thing is to find the formula that works for you. Experiment. Explore. Accept the inevitable frustration that will come if the method you first choose does not work well. Adopt a trial-and-error attitude, with the knowledge that you will eventually come upon a working equation.

Rome wasn't built in a day, and a good sleep regimen won't be built in a night. By understanding what keeps your brain alert and agitated, and then practicing methods for quieting your mind and letting go of your worries, you are taking the most important steps of the journey. The restful night of sleep you will ultimately find will top off your tank, balance your biochemistry, and leave you filled up in a way that will keep you from sneaking off to the cookie jar for energy and on track for losing weight.

YOUR PRESCRIPTION FOR REDUCING STRESS AND RESTORING YOUR SOUL

- Pick at least one stress-reduction exercise that will help you keep stress under control and quiet your mind at night.

- Each day, make time to restore your soul—via meditation, prayer, or any other means you choose to let go of worries, anxieties, and stressful thoughts and renew your mind and emotions.

- Schedule time each week to have fun. Do something that is truly enjoyable for you and forget about everything stressful during this time.

- Get away for a day or a weekend several times a year and do something relaxing. Take a one-week vacation at least once a year and get away from everything stressful, including telephones, e-mails, and anything else connected to work.

- Visit a health spa or get a massage occasionally.

- Practice appreciation and live from a thankful heart. It's a powerful way to combat stress.

CHAPTER FOUR

Step Three: Exercising for Better Sleep and a Slimmer You

Now that you're sleeping better and are a little more relaxed, Step Three is to exercise away those pounds! Think of this step as healthy and enjoyable movement, not as a chore. *Movement* is the key word, because our bodies are made to move. They are marvelously fashioned to walk, run, lift, jump, bend, stretch, work, play, and, finally, to lie down, rest, and drift naturally off to sleep. A healthy, trim, energetic, and vibrant body is a body that moves.

However, for many people, the natural inclination of the body to move has been lost through years of inactivity. We begin to think of the *joy* of movement as the *work* of exercise. And we don't do enough of it because we're tired from the stresses of daily life and the pressures of work and home. We sit down to rest, yet we do not feel rested. We lie down to sleep, but truly restorative sleep eludes us. The good news is that even a small amount of exercise, consistently and over time, gives huge rewards. Not only will we look and feel better, but we'll be nourished and strengthened—inside and out.

Movement builds strong muscles, bones, and connective tissue. And exercise creates a body that's trim and fit. Movement also has numerous benefits for the internal workings of our body. It strengthens our immune system, keeps our heart and cardiovascular system healthy, helps metabolize nutrients, builds new proteins and hormones, carries waste products out of our system, relieves stress, and enables our body to enter into a restful, peaceful sleep.

Many researchers are now studying the effects of exercise on sleep. They are documenting what may seem intuitively obvious: Getting a little exercise not only helps us lose weight and feel better, but also contributes significantly to a good night's sleep.

Ask just about any doctor, exercise physiologist, chiropractor, physical therapist, or anyone else in the health field and they will tell you that exercise is good for you. If you're physically able, even a slight increase in your level of movement will help you feel better, sleep better, and lose weight, particularly for those who have been leading a sedentary lifestyle. Just half an hour of moderate exercise, like a brisk walk, can be enough to help you sleep and improve your physical fitness.

A number of studies have been done on targeted groups who reported difficulty falling and staying asleep. The researchers found that increased exercise positively affected the ability of their subjects to sleep. Compared with control groups, they had improved general quality of sleep, quicker onset of sleep, and longer sleep duration, plus they generally felt more rested in the morning. Exercise routines in these studies used a combination of low-impact aerobics, such as brisk walking, and some resistance training. They found that as little as thirty to forty minutes four or more times per week was effective in helping increase restful sleep.

As we discussed earlier, muscle-relaxation techniques and breathing exercises are also beneficial in helping us sleep. There are several forms of slow movement, stretching, and deep-breathing exercises that can be done any time of day and will provide many of

THE BEST TIME TO EXERCISE

Not everyone agrees on the best time to exercise. Some studies suggest that mornings are best. Others say afternoon or right after dinner. Most agree that late-night exercise, particularly if it's too vigorous (such as intense running or resistance training), will keep you awake.

In a study at Seattle's Fred Hutchinson Cancer Research Center, only participants who exercised in the morning experienced the beneficial effects on sleep. Those who exercised in the evening actually had more trouble falling asleep.

One possible explanation as to why morning exercise helps sleep is that it may affect the body's circadian rhythms, which affect sleep quality. (Circadian rhythms are the patterns our body repeats in a twenty-four-hour cycle.) Morning exercise may get the body clock in alignment, and evening exercise may upset it. More research is needed to confirm this theory. However, we suggest that you do more strenuous exercises earlier in the day, or at least three hours before you go to bed, as these activities tend to rev up the metabolism and may keep you awake at night. The best evening exercises are those that involve stretching, relaxing, and breathing.

the benefits of more intense movement-oriented exercise. But that's just one of the many tips we'll give you in the following pages to help you find a variety of exercises that fit your lifestyle and are fun for you.

A study regarding the effects exercise has on sleep was presented at the American College of Sports Medicine's fiftieth annual meeting. The research showed that exercise has effects similar to sleeping pills, and indicated that people who have trouble sleeping should increase their daily activity levels.

Shawn D. Youngstedt, PhD, a sleep researcher at the University of California–San Diego, suggests that exercise has a beneficial effect on our circadian rhythms, which are the brain's natural way of telling us when to sleep and when to be active. Since exercise promotes shifts in the body clock, it could be effective in treating circadian-related sleep problems. Such problems are mostly associated with individuals whose body clocks are thrown off sync by working at odd or varying hours or traveling across time zones. He also suggests that exercising outdoors may provide added benefits, since light exposure has sleep-promoting and antidepressant effects.

Light, specifically full-spectrum light, positively affects the levels of serotonin and other neurotransmitters in our nervous system. Antidepressant drugs such as Prozac, Zoloft, and Paxil, which are known as selective serotonin reuptake inhibitors (SSRIs), affect these same pathways in our brain. If possible, it is far better to take frequent breaks and get some exercise outdoors than to take drugs. During the dark days of winter, use full-spectrum lightbulbs and supplement your diet with vitamin-D-rich foods such as cod-liver oil. The light must be taken in through your eyes, so artificial tanning beds will not benefit serotonin levels or increase your ability to sleep.

Another theory suggests that lack of physical activity contributes to insomnia by inhibiting the daily rise and fall of the body-temperature rhythm. This theory postulates that exercise improves sleep by producing a significant rise in body temperature, followed by a drop a few hours later. The drop in body temperature, which persists for two to four hours after exercise, makes it easier to fall asleep and stay asleep.

A study on sleep and exercise conducted in Finland found that 43 percent of the subjects who increased their exercise over a three-month period reported improved sleep, whereas 30 percent of the subjects who decreased their exercise over the same period reported poorer-quality or reduced-duration sleep. These results further support the notion that increased exercise leads to improved sleep.

Based on all these facts, it's time to get moving! There are literally hundreds of different ways to move and exercise your body to help you lose weight, feel great, and sleep restfully. Maybe you already have a favorite way of moving, but perhaps we can inspire you to move in ways you haven't tried before. Different movements are designed to achieve diverse results. The following suggestions are divided into three general categories: Aerobic Exercises, Weight and Resistance Training, and Stretching, Relaxing, and Breathing Exercises. For a balanced routine, choose one or two from each category to practice. Your initial goal is to do something three or more times throughout the week for about forty-five to sixty minutes at a time. Start slowly, but stay consistent. You will be delighted with the results!

AEROBIC EXERCISES

Aerobic literally means "in the presence of oxygen." Our bodies require oxygen in each cell for the production of energy. Aerobic activities are those designed to bring maximum energy into our cells through low-intensity, sustained movements that rely on oxygen for energy. These activities build endurance, burn fat, and condition the cardiovascular system.

Most studies regarding the effects of exercise on sleep recommend moderate exercise, such as low-impact aerobics or walking, performed a minimum of thirty to forty minutes three or more times a week. This prescription is perfect for those who have been living a sedentary lifestyle or who are just beginning to exercise. As you progress in your exercise program, you will probably want to increase the time and intensity of your workout, perhaps adding a few of the activities outlined below. Go slowly at first, and remember that it's consistent exercise over time that yields the greatest results. Check with your doctor if you have any health concerns, then start moving; you can increase your time and intensity later.

Aerobic exercise is an ideal way to dissipate the excess energy that builds up if you're living a high-stress lifestyle or simply sitting too much. Rather than eating more food, drinking more coffee, taking drugs, tapping your toes, fidgeting, biting your nails, or yelling at your spouse or co-workers, why not take an exercise break? It is far more effective and healthy to channel pent-up emotions and excess energy into an active, aerobic form of exercise.

Aerobic activities such as walking, jogging, swimming, bicycling, racquet sports, skiing, step aerobics, and dancing are great for weight loss and promote better sleep. Find something you enjoy doing so your exercise is a delight, not a chore; otherwise, you'll end up creating more stress than you already have. Try a variety of exercises, and choose something that feels good to you. A number of possibilities are listed below, but there are certainly dozens of other aerobic activities you can try. Just keep moving a little every day and you will begin to sleep better. Best of all, you'll build muscle and rev up your metabolism so that you'll burn more calories, even at a resting heart rate, and thus you'll begin to lose weight, look more toned, and feel great!

Walking

Walking is an exercise that practically everyone can do. It's simple, you can do it almost anywhere, including indoors, and it's an effective way to lose weight and improve your sleep. Walking at a brisk pace will keep you in the midrange of aerobic activity and won't put a strain on your joints and ligaments the way many more vigorous forms of aerobic activity can.

Walking, like most forms of movement, increases your sense of well-being. The increased level of activity aids sleep because it helps you fall asleep more quickly and spend more time in the deeper stages of sleep, known as slow-wave—the phase of sleep that helps restore the body, and the stage where you wake up less often.

Some of the benefits of walking include reducing stress, loosening tight muscles, and lessening the symptoms of depression and anxiety. Because walking helps you sleep, you'll feel renewed and refreshed enough to keep moving the next day, thus breaking the negative cycle of tiredness, which keeps you from exercising and makes you more tired and less able to sleep. Taking a brisk walk every day can turn this upside down.

The following ideas will assist you in getting started with a consistent walking program:

- Go slowly at first. Find a pace that's right for you. Walk as far and as long as is comfortable, working up to longer, brisker walks. Give your body time to get used to the increased demand, but try to push yourself just a little extra each day.

- Take a short walk before or after dinner to relax your nervous system and at the same time burn some calories. The use of energy combined with the release of stress relaxes your body and mind and will help you sleep better and longer.

- Find a friend to walk with for companionship and motivation. Dogs are great walking partners, too. If you don't have a dog to walk, perhaps you can borrow one from a friend or neighbor. Your canine friend will keep you moving and help you focus on the simple things of life, like the smell of flowers.

- Walk briskly enough to break a sweat, but not so fast that you run out of breath. Begin to slow down toward the end of your walk, as this will bring your heartbeat down to its resting rate, which prepares your body for a decent night's sleep.

An excellent resource book on the benefits of walking is Leslie Sansone's *Walk Away the Pounds* program. On days when you can't get outside, try Leslie's *In Home Walking* series on video or DVD. Her book and video or DVD can be purchased at www.lesliesansonevideos.com.

Rebounding

Rebounding is an exercise performed on a mini trampoline, which is also appropriately called a rebounder. It is fun, easy to do, safe, and very effective. You can use it in the comfort of your own home—no need to pound the pavement, dodge dogs or cars, or put up with bad weather. One proponent claims, "Rebound exercise is the most efficient and effective exercise yet devised by man." It's also one of our personal favorites, since we live in a rainy climate and have a busy schedule—a few minutes of rebounding in the morning gets us up and going for the day.

Rebounding is a zero-impact aerobic exercise that improves blood circulation and increases the capacity of both the heart and lungs. It's also one of the most effective exercises for moving the fluids of the lymphatic system, which carries waste products out of the body. With regular rebounding, the resting heart rate can decline ten beats per minute, which means five thousand fewer heartbeats in a single night's sleep.

Rebounding protects the joints from damage, as your body is subjected to gravitational pulls ranging from zero at the top of each bounce to two to three times the force of gravity at the bottom, depending on how high you're rebounding. Unlike jogging on hard surfaces, which puts extreme stress on certain joints such as the ankles and knees, eventually damaging them, rebounding affects every joint and cell in the body equally and does not put extra stress on certain areas of the body.

As noted, one of the greatest advantages of rebounding is its effect on the lymph system, which carries nutrients to all the cells of our body and carries waste products away. Vigorous exercise such as rebounding can increase lymph flow by fifteen to thirty times. Because lymph is totally dependent on physical exercise (or lymphatic drainage massage) to move, without adequate movement the lymph system cannot properly excrete toxic waste products, which affects the cells, limiting their ability to efficiently absorb life-giving nutrients. This situation contributes to a general sluggishness, and can eventually lead to degenerative diseases such as heart disease, cancer, and arthritis, as well as early aging. It can also keep you awake at night with effects of toxicity, including aching muscles, headache, a general sense of malaise, or depression.

Why is rebounding so good for the lymphatic system? There is no active lymph pump to move fluid through the lymph vessels the way our heart pumps blood through the blood vessels. The lymph system is passive, not active, and its vessels have valves that move fluid in one direction only. Therefore, active movement is required to keep the fluids moving. The main lymph vessels run up the legs, arms, and torso, so the vertical up-and-down movement of rebounding is especially effective at pumping lymph through them.

Rebounding has many other health-enhancing benefits, as well. For example, it is good for promoting deeper and easier relaxation and sleep. It allows the resting heart to beat less often. In addition, it helps manage body composition and improves muscle-to-fat ratio. It improves resting metabolic rate so that more calories are burned for hours after exercise. It circulates more oxygen to the tissues and causes muscles to move fluids through the body, lightening the heart's load. It strengthens the heart and other muscles in the body so that they work more efficiently. It lowers circulating cholesterol and triglyceride levels and enhances digestion and elimination processes.

The best way to begin rebounding is to bounce very slowly, keeping your feet in contact with the surface of the rebounder while your body moves up and down. After a few minutes, you will feel the energy moving through your limbs and up into your head. Even this gentle, slow movement will give you all the benefits of rebounding while strengthening the entire body. As your strength and balance increase, you can begin to bounce higher and faster. You can rebound while listening to music, watching television, or even talking on the phone. One of our favorites is to put on some old-time rock and roll and jump to the music. There are also tapes available on rebounding techniques if you want to get more serious about it.

You can wear running shoes or jump with bare feet; just make sure that what you have on your feet, such as socks, won't make you slip. Start with five minutes of rebounding and increase your time as fitness improves. If you are older or have been sedentary for a while, start with one or two minutes ten times per day, with at least thirty minutes between sessions. It's important to gradually build up your time, especially if you're older or out of shape, as the only contraindication to rebounding is the possibility of prolapsed organs. This can be avoided by starting slowly and rebounding more often, which allows time to strengthen the connective tissues around the internal organs.

IF YOU HAVE PHYSICAL LIMITATIONS

If you have physical limitations or disabilities, consider using a rebounder, a lymphasizer, or a pool for a safe workout.

Rebounder. Inactive or wheelchair-bound people, or those with joint problems who have not been able to exercise, often find that rebounding gives them renewed vigor and zest for life. Blind or handicapped people can purchase a handrail that attaches to the rebounder. Hyperactive children are reported to calm down after a few days of rebounding. Rebounding is for everyone. You can use the rebounder mini trampoline whenever you have a few minutes during the day.

Lymphasizer. The lymphasizer, also known as the healthy swinger, is an ideal alternative or a great addition to an exercise regimen because it will actively move lymph and blood through your body when you lie down on it. It's very beneficial for those with circulation problems in their feet that stem from such issues as diabetes or steroid usage. With this machine, you can have a low-impact workout that requires no active movement. You just lie on the floor with your feet in the grooves and get the aerobic benefits of half an hour of exercise in only ten minutes.

The lymphasizer provides a simple exercise without applying any stress on the spine or other body parts. As you lie down on the floor with your feet in the grooves of the machine your body will rock from side to side like the movement of a fish. This simple rocking motion maintains a proper energy balance and oxygen supply to the body. Regular use of this relaxing massage movement stimulates your body and achieves relaxation and stress reduction. A sense of well-being is immediately noticeable from the massaging swing action. Using the lymphasizer before bedtime promotes more restful sleep as well as weight loss.

Though this machine is great for everyone, it can be excellent for the disabled, for anyone with hip, knee, or ankle problems, for those who are very overweight and find other forms of exercise difficult, or for those who for other medical reasons are unable to even bounce slowly on a rebounder.

Swimming or water aerobics. Water exercise is another good alternative for those who have access to a pool. It's an excellent way to exercise without putting stress on the joints, which makes it a good choice for anyone with hip, knee, or ankle problems, or for the very overweight who need to start exercising without damaging their joints. You can begin by holding on to the side of the pool and kicking or moving your arms and legs. Another suggestion is to simply walk slowly back and forth across the shallow end of the pool. The increased resistance of the water will help strengthen your muscles without putting any strain on your joints and ligaments.

Fast Walking, Jogging, and Running

Fast walking, jogging, or running is the next step up to a higher fitness level. The basic idea is to get your heart working hard enough to propel you into greater cardiovascular fitness. Gradually increasing the intensity of your workout by speeding up your pace will push your body out of its comfort zone and help you lose weight more quickly. Try increasing your pace until you are uncomfortable for a minute, then fall back to your usual pace. Fast walking, jogging, or running can be done outside, or inside on a treadmill. One great advantage of the treadmill is that you can increase the incline so you burn more calories while maintaining the same pace.

Fast walking puts less stress on your body than running, especially on your knees and ankles, and if you do it fast and far enough—five miles per hour for forty-five minutes or more—it can get you just as fit as running or jogging. If you have the time, walking at slower speeds for an hour or more will also burn the maximum amount of fat. High-energy walking styles, such as racewalking, are better than running for building strength in your arms and torso and streamlining flabby thighs.

Running has most of the same benefits as walking, but dedicated runners also report the well-known runner's high, which results from the release of endorphins. The brain's "feel-good" neurotransmitters, endorphins have pain-relieving properties similar to morphine.

Fast walking, jogging, or running regularly has also been proven to help fight the aging process. It prevents muscle and bone loss that often occur with age. Our bones are made to accommodate whatever demands are placed upon them. By sitting at a desk or computer all day, many of us allow our bones to grow weaker, but running regularly puts on our skeleton the demands it needs to stay healthy. In addition to keeping our internal organs from aging quickly, regular high-intensity exercise, like running, has also been proven to promote release of human growth hormone (GH), which promotes weight loss and better sleep.

Fast walking or running helps fight disease because it strengthens the heart, maintains the elasticity of the arteries, and lowers blood pressure, thus reducing the risk of hypertension, stroke, and heart attack. During aerobic activity, our arteries expand and contract nearly three times as much as usual.

Fast walking, jogging, and running also help maintain and improve general health by raising HDL (the "good" cholesterol), reducing the risk of blood clots, and encouraging the use of the 50 percent of our lungs that usually goes unused. These activities boost the immune system by creating a higher concentration of lymphocytes—the white blood cells that attack infection.

A study by John Trinder, PhD, and colleagues in Australia compared the sleep habits of trained distance runners (an average of forty-five miles per week), serious weight lifters (twelve hours per week), and sedentary folks. The runners fell asleep more quickly after going to bed and experienced a longer duration of deep sleep than the individuals in the other two groups. In other words, the runners had greater sleep efficiency, which is the ratio of the amount of time you are asleep to the total amount of time you are in bed.

During running, sympathetic nervous system activity increases, but endurance training leads to a decrease in sympathetic activity relative to parasympathetic activity when we're not exercising. The sympathetic (SNS) and parasympathetic (PNS) nervous systems are part of the autonomic nervous system. The SNS activates the fight-or-flight response, which activates the secretion of adrenaline. The PNS serves to slow heart rate, increase intestinal and gland activity, and relax the sphincter muscles. This alteration in the balance of sympathetic to parasympathetic activity may allow us to fall asleep more quickly and to sleep more deeply. Running too close to bedtime, however, can leave the SNS stimulated for several hours, making it more difficult to fall asleep.

Cycling

Cycling is an excellent aerobic conditioner if it is done with enough intensity and for a long enough time. In other words, just coasting around the neighborhood on your bicycle will not get your heart working hard enough. Sustained cycling, however, will build strength in your back and legs, increase your endurance, and help reduce stress. Depending on the speed and terrain, it can burn 350 to 450 calories an hour or more.

Cycling produces less stress on the body than running. It is an excellent choice for anyone who is unable to run or do other activities because of orthopedic problems, overweight, or other conditions that are aggravated by weight-bearing exercises.

Outdoor biking is fun in summer or in warmer climates, but not when the weather is cold, rainy, windy, or icy. The alternative for biking enthusiasts is the many kinds of indoor stationary bikes, which can keep you just as fit. Most health clubs also offer stationary bikes and cycling classes (spinning), which increase motivation in most people.

Swimming

Swimming is a great activity. It tones your entire body while providing an excellent cardiovascular workout; it strengthens your heart muscle and improves delivery of oxygen to muscles throughout your body. Swimming is also relaxing and can thus contribute to improved sleep.

It's hard to beat swimming when it comes to a sport that builds the body, soothes the mind, regulates breathing, stimulates circulation, and puts no stress on the joints. That's why it's an ideal exercise for just about everyone—the old, the young, overweight people, people with hip, knee, and ankle problems, and active people with no health problems at all. Plus, swimming has a calorie-burning potential of 350 to 420 calories per hour, so it's great for weight loss. The obvious disadvantage is that you need a pool, which is not always an option.

Aerobics—Step, Nonstep, and Dance Aerobics

Many people enjoy working out with others in a class setting because it stimulates them, is fun, encourages them to push harder than they would on their own, and has a set time when they must show up—which is often more motivating than a self-determined schedule. Almost every gym and health club has one or several aerobics classes to choose from: step aerobics, nonstep aerobics, dance aerobic classes, and total-body workout classes that combine light weights with lots of movement for an aerobic benefit. Find a class that you like and go for it! Total-body workout is one of my favorites. I can personally testify that it is one of the quickest ways to get in shape.

WEIGHT AND RESISTANCE TRAINING

Weight-bearing exercises such as strength training with machines and/or free weights are one of the most efficient ways to develop muscle strength and muscle tone by increasing lean body mass, which is important for individuals attempting weight loss. These exercises strengthen the bones and connective tissues, thus helping to prevent injuries and osteoporosis. They also help develop coordination and balance.

Weight training forces your body to produce more muscle. As a result, your body increases the size and number of the mitochondria it produces. Mitochondria are the cell organelles that burn glucose and produce energy. They are found in high concentrations in heart and skeletal muscles, which require large amounts of energy for mechanical work; in the pancreas, where there is biosynthesis; and in the kidneys, where the process of excretion begins. They can be called cellular furnaces, because this is where nutrients from the food we eat are burned to produce ATP, which produces cellular energy for the work of the body.

PILATES: STRETCHING AND STRENGTHENING

Pilates is a series of exercises designed to improve flexibility and strength through a variety of stretching and balancing movements. It was developed by Joseph Pilates, a prisoner of war during World War II, and has become increasingly popular in the last several years. Pilates introduced his exercises to inmates of a German internment camp, helping them keep physically fit. He also introduced mat workout and physical exercise equipment made from bedsprings.

Today Pilates has become particularly popular among dancers, athletes, celebrities, and models, because in addition to helping develop flexibility without causing a strain on the muscles, it also improves posture and gives people a longer, leaner appearance. A regular Pilates regimen results in a flatter stomach, a thinner waist, and leaner thighs, as well as increasing mobility in joints. Pilates helps improve strength, tone, flexibility, and balance, and makes the body less prone to injury. It reduces stress, relieves tension, and boosts energy through deep stretching.

Chiropractic doctors recommend Pilates for strengthening the back and the spine. Physiotherapists also recommend Pilates to those seeking rehabilitation after injuries to their limbs. Pilates is recommended for everyone—the young, the elderly, sedentary people, those who suffer from osteoporosis, and people who are overweight. According to Joseph Pilates, the correct practice of Pilates mat work, along with proper nutrition and sleep, will also result in wellness and a sense of well-being.

Resistance training, or weight training, increases strength, builds and tones muscles, and increases muscular endurance. It also helps you develop self-confidence and body satisfaction because you can begin to look better and leaner after only a few short weeks of a concentrated program.

No matter how old, weak, or out of shape you are, you can boost your strength and improve the way you look and feel by getting involved with a sensible weight-training program. People over forty who have not been active, or who have high blood pressure, heart disease, back pain, arthritis, or any other health problems, will want to check with their doctor before beginning any kind of strength-training program.

Weight training is a terrific anti-aging program because it counteracts the natural tendency of the body to grow weaker as it ages. Weight-bearing exercise is an important component in osteoporosis prevention. Without some kind of regular strength training, we can lose up to half a pound of muscle every year after age twenty-five. With weight training, we stay stronger longer and look leaner and more toned, too. If you've ever been to a gym with serious weight-training programs, you will see men and women in their fifties, sixties, even seventies and sometimes eighties who look as trim and fit as a twenty-five-year-old. This should encourage you to add some form of strength training to your regular routine.

STRETCHING, RELAXING, AND BREATHING EXERCISES

Throughout history, many cultures have devised exercises that are designed to strengthen and stretch the body while relaxing and focusing the mind. Some of these techniques are accompanied by elaborate philosophies, yet the simple essence of their techniques is to stretch and relax the muscles, plus control breathing so that more

RELAXATION BREATHING EXERCISE

1. Lie down flat on your back with your arms at your sides, palms up. Close your eyes and take a couple of deep breaths.

2. Continue breathing deeply and evenly through both nostrils for a few moments. Breathe all the way to the bottom of your lungs, then let your abdomen rise as the breath enters (don't try to hold your tummy in). As you exhale, let any remaining tension in your body flow out with your breath.

3. Visualize a peaceful and relaxing scene. Begin to focus on the right side of your body. Focus first on your fingers, then your hand and your arm. Tense the muscles in your right arm and hand by clenching your hand into a tight fist. Release and let the tension flow from your fingertips up your arm to your shoulder. Breathe it out.

4. Repeat on the left side of your body, moving from your fingers, up your arm, and into your shoulder, breathing slowly as you do.

5. Now focus on your shoulders. Tense your shoulder blades and then relax them three times.

6. Focus on your feet, first on the right side of your body, then on the left. Tense and release your toes, then flex your feet hard. As you relax them, feel all the tension drain from your feet, ankles, calves, knees, thighs, buttocks, and abdomen. Breathe out any remaining tension.

7. Turn your head to the right and left, relaxing any tension in your neck muscles, and then let your neck totally relax as you continue breathing. Finally, tense the muscles of your face. Be aware of and release any tension around your jaw, mouth, eyes, nose, ears, forehead, or scalp. Let the tension go as you continue to breathe slowly and rhythmically.

8. Stay in this relaxed state for a few minutes, letting the floor support you. Focus on your breathing, releasing all other concerns. Let your breath come from deep in your abdomen, and let it flow smoothly and slowly.

This simple exercise is a way of telling your mind and body that it is now permissible for it to relax and to stop thinking, working, and struggling.

It's important not to be hard on yourself. Don't judge whether you're doing the sleep relaxation perfectly. Simply by attempting this exercise, you will begin to calm and relax your body. Each time you do it, you'll find yourself entering more quickly into a peaceful state. You will begin to look forward to this time of relaxation.

oxygen is delivered into the cells, especially the brain, thus calming and relaxing the whole body.

Stretching and relaxation exercises can increase suppleness, enhance mental and physical relaxation, and improve the quality of your sleep. Stretching is something everyone can do, no matter their age or level of ability. Gentle movements, deep breathing, and long stretches are ideal methods of relaxation to help us sleep. The combination of stretching, relaxing, and breathing promotes a slowing down of the body and mind and encourages sleep. The body is not overstimulated, as it may be if some of the more strenuous exercises are performed late in the day. Therefore, these techniques are an excellent choice for those whose schedule allows for exercise only after work or in the evening.

The advantage of stretching is that it strengthens the nervous system, thus relieving stress and anxiety. It also strengthens and relaxes the skeletal, muscular, digestive, cardiovascular, and glandular systems, thus calming the body and mind.

One theory about how breathing and relaxation affect our ability to sleep comes from ayurvedic medicine, an ancient healing science developed in India. This theory claims that all disease is caused by indigestion. If we have poor digestion—at any level in our physical, mental, or emotional beings—we haven't completely extracted what is helpful and eliminated what is indigestible.

Experts tell us that stretching, relaxation, and breathing exercises will improve the quality of sleep because of their beneficial effect on the nervous system, and in particular the brain. This results from the increased blood supply to the brain, which has the effect of normalizing the sleep cycle. You will need less sleep because of the improved quality of your sleep, and also because these exercises increase the elimination of toxins from the body.

To unwind mentally and physically as you prepare to sleep, begin by breathing deeply and rhythmically for five to ten minutes. This will allow you to slow down from the activities of the day.

Next, do some gentle stretches for ten to fifteen minutes. Go slowly and listen to your body. Don't try to stretch too far at first. Try holding a stretch for the count of twenty-five; relax and breathe. Then try the same stretch again, this time reaching farther into it. Each time you do the movement, you will get a slightly better stretch.

Finally, use relaxation breathing exercises. You can try the exercise in this chapter (page 97) or the one on page 53 in Chapter 3.

YOUR PRESCRIPTION FOR EXERCISES TO SLEEP WELL AND LOSE WEIGHT

- Pick one form of aerobic exercise that you will do at least three times a week.
- Pick one method of strength training that you can incorporate into your regimen each week.
- Choose a stretching/breathing routine that you will include every week in your exercise program.

CHAPTER FIVE

Step Four: The Optimum Diet for Sound Sleep and Super Weight Loss

We all know that what we put in our mouth affects our waistline. What we may not realize is that what we eat also affects our sleep, which plays a key role in our weight loss efforts. Since the all-important good night's sleep can be affected positively or negatively by what you put in your mouth, taking control of your body's biochemistry so you can sleep well helps balance your hormones, enabling you to control your blood sugar so that it's not too high or too low. This helps you manage your hunger and food cravings and helps prevent leptin and insulin resistance.

One of the keys to a restful night's sleep is to calm your mind and body rather than rev it up. Certain foods contribute to restful sleep, while others stir up energy and keep you awake. Some foods are calming, such as those containing tryptophan—an amino acid the body uses to make serotonin, the neurotransmitter that slows down nerve traffic so your brain isn't so busy at night.

Other foods, like those that contain caffeine or sugar, energize the mind and body by producing neurochemicals that perk up the brain.

Certain foods, drinks, supplements, and medications may be responsible for your ability (or lack thereof) to sleep well by increasing hormonal activity or by reversing or compounding the effects of tension or anxiety. Therefore, it's important to choose your foods and drinks wisely so you can sleep more restfully. In so doing, you can turn off the hormones that send the *Eat more food—make more fat* message.

This practical dietary advice is the fourth and final step of the Sleep Away the Pounds Program. It's simply all about making wise dietary choices that will enable your body to relax, drift off to sleep easily, and stay asleep throughout the night. It's also about training your body to burn more fat than sugar, balancing your blood sugar metabolism, and preventing insulin and leptin resistance. It's interesting to note that the foods that help you sleep well are also the foods that help you lose weight. And the foods that keep you from getting a good night's sleep are usually the ones that pack on the pounds. In the pages that follow, you'll find tips for making the best food choices, along with the foods you should avoid and the supplements that can help you sleep well and lose weight—all so you can jump-start your metabolism and start sleeping off the pounds.

FOODS THAT HELP YOU SLEEP WELL

Though foods are not drugs, and they won't necessarily make you drop off to dreamland as soon as your head hits the pillow, certain foods can help you relax and sleep better throughout the night.

Celery has a calming effect. It contains silicon, which strengthens nerve and heart tissue.

Chia and jujube seeds have a sedative effect. In Chinese medicine, these seeds are thought to nourish the heart and calm the spirit.

Dark green (chlorophyll-rich) vegetables help promote restful sleep.

Lettuce and lettuce juice. During World War II, a compound in lettuce called lactucarium was used as a sedative for soldiers. All lettuces possess some of this substance. Prickly lettuce and wild lettuce have the most, but the common garden lettuce does contain it, too. Mixed with a little lemon juice for flavor, lettuce juice is an effective sleep-inducing drink. Lettuce juice has been used for restlessness, sleeplessness, and hysteria in children.

Mulberries are used in Chinese medicine for improving insomnia by calming the mind.

Oysters are used in Chinese medicine for improving insomnia.

Tryptophan-rich foods. Have you ever noticed that you're ready to fall asleep not long after the Thanksgiving Day turkey dinner? Part of that effect is certainly due to eating more than usual, and a varied mixture at that. It's the abundance of tryptophan in turkey, how-ever, that most diet-minded folks say produces the desire to slumber. Tryptophan is an amino acid that is a precursor of the sleep-inducing substances serotonin and melatonin—in other words, it's the raw material that the brain uses to build relaxing neurotransmitters. Making more tryptophan available by eating foods that contain this substance and making sure that more tryptophan gets to the brain will help make you sleepy. On the other hand, nutrients such as the amino acid tyrosine that make tryptophan less available can disturb sleep.

Foods rich in tryptophan include turkey, milk, cottage cheese, chicken, eggs, and nuts, particularly almonds. Compared with other amino acids, tryptophan is found only in small quantities, so you may need a little more of these foods than others. Also, tryptophan metabolism depends on the balance of other amino acids in the bloodstream. Eating a high-protein meal with complex carbohydrates such as vegetables is a good idea; otherwise, it may keep you awake, since protein-rich foods also contain the amino acid tyrosine, which perks up the brain.

TRYPTOPHAN-RICH FOODS

- Dairy products: cottage cheese, cheese, milk, yogurt
- Seafood
- Meat
- Poultry, especially turkey
- Whole grains
- Beans
- Rice
- Hummus
- Lentils
- Nuts: almonds, hazelnuts, peanuts
- Eggs
- Sesame seeds, sunflower seeds

We've found it helpful to keep sliced turkey and raw almonds on hand for times when we wake up and can't get back to sleep. Try eating a few bites of a tryptophan-rich food if you awaken in the night; also, take a vitamin B_6 and magnesium supplement to ensure that the tryptophan is converted to serotonin. Niacin may also be helpful in that it moves tryptophan metabolism toward formation of serotonin.

Vegetables and other complex carbohydrates. Tryptophan and carbohydrates work together to relax your body. When the amino acids tryptophan and tyrosine arrive at the brain cells, you'll want more tryptophan to enter. If more tyrosine enters the brain cells, neuroactivity will rev up. If more tryptophan gets in, the brain will calm down. If you eat complex carbohydrates such as vegetables or brown rice with protein for your evening meal, insulin will be released to deal with carbohydrates in the bloodstream. Insulin keeps tyrosine at bay, allowing the brain-calming tryptophan effect to be higher than that of the brain-revving tyrosine. It's also wise to include calcium, which helps the brain use the tryptophan to manufacture melatonin.

Virgin coconut oil. Though virgin coconut oil can keep you awake if you eat very much of it late in the day, due to its energizing qualities, many people have found that it does help them sleep better when consumed during the day. You should be able to use it for cooking dinner without creating the revving-up effects. The best part is that virgin coconut oil is slimming; it's dominated by the medium-chain triglycerides that the liver likes to burn, which helps you lose weight. We've devoted an entire book to this subject called *The Coconut Diet*, which will give you great recipes for how to incorporate it into your diet.

Whole grains. Brown rice and oats, in particular, have a calming, soothing effect on the nervous system and the mind. Complex carbohydrates such as these also boost serotonin, which promotes better sleep.

NUTRITIONAL SUPPLEMENTS THAT CAN HELP YOU SLEEP BETTER

There are a number of nutritional supplements that will help you sleep better and some that facilitate weight loss. Following is a list of nutrients that you may find helpful for your Sleep Away the Pounds Program.

Amino Acids

GABA (gamma-aminobutyric acid), glutamine, and glycine are inhibitory amino acids (neurotransmitters) that act directly on the limbic system. GABA calms the brain and helps shut down the emotionally loaded limbic system. Glutamine helps balance the brain. Glycine helps to regulate stress levels.

GABA acts as a neurotransmitter, relaying information from one cell to another. GABA acts particularly well in the limbic system to calm the body. When the limbic system is hyperexcited and anxiety, fear, panic, or other negative emotions start running the show, GABA restores balance by occupying receptor sites that turn down the "emotional alarm system."

You may have taken the edge off your emotions with a cocktail, a glass of wine, a beer, or a tranquilizer, which all work by attaching to these receptor sites. But there are a host of problems associated with these calming substances, such as addiction, liver congestion or damage, and poor sleep. GABA has none of the drug side effects and can also be used for situational anxiety such as public speaking or flying as well as for insomnia.

Phosphatidylserine is an amino acid that helps the brain regulate the amount of cortisol produced by the adrenals. It is helpful for those who cannot sleep because of high cortisol levels, which are most often induced by stress. Cortisol is usually produced at high levels in the morning to awaken the body, but it's often found to be high at night in people with high stress levels, which prevents them from falling asleep or causes them to awaken during the night. Supplementation: 100 mg daily as needed.

Supplementation: To relieve anxiety, take 500 to 750 mg GABA as needed. For insomnia, take 500 mg an hour before bedtime. Note, however, that if you are relatively healthy and eat a very nutritious diet, these amino acids may be too powerful for your system. Still, if you're an emotionally charged person, GABA, in particular, may be quite helpful in calming your mind and emotions.

Calcium

A deficiency of calcium can cause you to wake up in the middle of the night and not be able to get back to sleep; it can also cause restlessness. Low calcium leads to muscles that stay contracted and can't relax, and it may cause leg cramps during the night. Calcium helps the brain use the amino acid tryptophan to manufacture melatonin. It has also been shown to help people lose weight. Best food sources include kale, dulse, collard and turnip greens, almonds, parsley, corn tortillas (with lime), dandelion greens, Brazil nuts, watercress, goat's milk, tofu, sunflower seeds, yogurt, buckwheat, sesame seeds, ripe olives, and broccoli.

Supplementation: Calcium citrate and liquid calcium are the best forms. The recommended dosage is 1,200 to 1,500 mg daily, divided in doses with meals, with 500 mg taken forty-five minutes before bedtime.

Conjugated Linoleic Acid (CLA)

CLA is a fatty acid found in high amounts in naturally raised, grass-fed beef and lamb and dairy fat. Grain-fed animals have very low levels of CLA compared with grass-fed. Though there's no promise you'll sleep better by consuming CLA, research does indicate you'll increase fat burning while you sleep. A study published in the December 2000 issue of the *Journal of Nutrition* found that CLA encourages muscle growth while simultaneously promoting fat loss by decreasing the amount of fat stored in fat cells, raising metabolism, and burning fat—all while you get a good night's sleep. In a separate study conducted at Purdue University in Indiana, CLA was found to improve insulin levels in about two-thirds of diabetic patients, and moderately reduced blood glucose levels and triglyceride levels. It has also been shown to lower insulin resistance and to decrease abdominal fat. (Adrenal imbalances and hormonal shifts can cause rapid buildup of abdominal fat.) Your best food choices are grass-fed, organically raised beef, lamb, and dairy products.

Supplementation: The recommended dosage is 3.4 grams per day, taken throughout the day. CLA needs to be taken consistently for several months, however, before you see results.

Chromium

Chromium can be helpful if you have a blood sugar imbalance. People with low blood sugar (hypoglycemia) can benefit from this supplement, because they may wake up in the middle of the night if their blood sugar gets too low. Brewer's yeast is a good source of chromium. Other food sources include oysters, potatoes, eggs, and chicken.

Supplementation: Chromium picolinate is the best supplemental form. The recommended dosage is 250 mcg twice a day.

Copper

A deficiency of copper can contribute to insomnia. US Department of Agriculture (USDA) researchers at the Human Nutrition Research Center in Grand Forks, North Dakota, report that women who are deficient in copper and iron are more likely to have problems sleeping. Based on these findings, James C. Penland, PhD, of the department's Agricultural Research Service, notes that while there are many reasons for insomnia, inadequate consumption of certain essential trace minerals, particularly copper, for an extended period may be a contributing factor. When eleven women in the copper study received only 0.8 mg of copper daily—less than half the 2 to 3 mg per day considered adequate—they slept for a longer period of time, but had difficulty getting to sleep and awoke feeling less rested than when they got an additional 2 mg per day. According to the 1985 food consumption figures from the USDA's Human Nutrition Information Service, the average copper intake for women ages nineteen to fifty is half the amount currently considered adequate. Most people get about 1 mg of copper a day. That is not enough of a deficiency to cause obvious symptoms, but it may be enough to affect sleep. The best food choices for copper are oysters, nuts, split peas, cod-liver oil, lamb chops, and butter.

Supplementation: The recommended dosage is 2 to 3 mg daily.

Iron

A deficiency of iron can contribute to insomnia. One study by the USDA found that women who got only one-third of the recommended dietary allowance (RDA) for iron experienced more awakenings during the night and poorer sleep quality than those who got the full RDA. The RDA for menstruating women is 15 mg; 10 mg is recommended for nonmenstruating women and men. Your best food choices are red meat, seeds, nuts, dark leafy greens, and seafood. Include vitamin C or vitamin-C-rich foods when you eat iron-rich foods, to enhance iron's absorption. Supplemental iron is not recommended, since iron supplements have been associated with cancer.

Magnesium

Magnesium is involved in hundreds of enzymatic reactions and numerous processes in the body, including digestion, energy production, muscle relaxation, and functions of the heart, adrenals, kidneys, brain, and nervous system. "Magnesium deficiency is actually fairly common; however, it is usually not looked for, and therefore not found or corrected," says Elson M. Haas, MD. A deficiency of magnesium will cause you to wake up after a few hours of sleep and not be able to drift off to sleep again.

Other signs and symptoms of magnesium deficiency include

fatigue, headaches, anxiousness, nervousness, backaches, mental confusion, irritability, weakness, heart disturbances, muscle cramps, and a predisposition to stress.

Interestingly, stress can cause depletion of magnesium levels. In a study of 165 boys, it was found that those with symptoms of depression, schizophrenia, and sleep disturbances had lower levels of magnesium in the blood. Calcium and magnesium produce calming effects on the brain, and magnesium also facilitates calcium absorption. Diuretic drugs, alcohol, tobacco, caffeine, sugar, soft water, and a high-carbohydrate, high-sodium, or high-calcium diet will cause magnesium loss, along with conditions such as low thyroid, diabetes, and chronic pain.

Magnesium-rich foods such as kelp, wheat bran and germ, tofu, beet greens, coconut, spinach, brown rice, almonds, and cashews can help induce sleep.

Supplementation: Magnesium citrate and liquid magnesium are the best forms; recommended dosage is 350 mg daily for men and 280 for women, with 250 mg of these amounts taken before bedtime. Therapeutic levels of magnesium used by physicians are commonly in the range of 600 to 1,000 mg. Calcium and magnesium taken forty-five minutes before bedtime have a tranquilizing effect. Use a two-to-one ratio, such as 500 mg of calcium and 250 mg of magnesium. Magnesium requires an acidic stomach environment for best absorption, so taking it between meals and at bedtime is recommended. *Note: If you have heart or kidney problems, be sure to consult your doctor before taking magnesium supplements.*

The B-Complex Vitamins

It is usually best to get your B vitamins in a complex. Though they are noted separately below, and from time to time you may need a little extra of one particular B vitamin, in the long term it's best to take a B-complex vitamin. The various B vitamins are all available in the appropriate amounts in these supplements, and can work synergistically together.

Niacinamide (vitamin B$_3$) is helpful for sleep-maintenance insomnia—when you awaken in the night and can't get back to sleep. Best food sources are brewer's yeast, peanuts, meat, poultry, and fish. (Niacinamide is the nonflush type.)

Supplementation: The recommended dosage is 100 mg to 1 gram at bedtime.

Pantothenic acid (vitamin B$_5$) deficiency can cause insomnia. To prevent a deficiency, eat foods rich in pantothenic acid such as brewer's yeast, liver, peanuts, mushrooms, split peas, perch, pecans, eggs, oatmeal, buckwheat, sunflower seeds, lentils, rye, and salmon.

Supplementation: 25 mcg of vitamin B$_{12}$ with 100 mg of pantothenic acid can serve as an effective anti-insomnia vitamin regimen.

Vitamin B$_1$(thiamin) works with niacin and vitamin B$_2$ to produce serotonin from tryptophan. Best food sources include brewer's yeast, wheat germ, sunflower seeds, pine nuts, peanuts, Brazil nuts, pecans, pinto and red beans, split peas, millet, wheat bran, pistachio nuts, navy beans, and buckwheat.

Supplementation: The recommended dosage is 50 to 100 mg daily.

Vitamin B$_6$ (pyridoxine) helps prevent insomnia. It is a needed co-factor to activate amino acids that help you sleep. It's also known to help people remember their dreams. Brewer's yeast is an excellent source of B vitamins, and is particularly rich in B$_6$. You can stir it into several ounces of juice. Other good food sources include seeds and nuts, fish (salmon, trout, mackerel), beans, lentils, split peas, and avocados.

Supplementation: The recommended dosage is 50 to 100 mg daily.

Inositol enhances REM sleep.

Supplementation: 100 mg daily, at bedtime.

5-Hydroxytryptophan (5-HTP)

This modified amino acid forms the neurotransmitter serotonin, which enhances mood and satiety and promotes relaxation. Along with melatonin, 5-HTP helps regulate sleep patterns. A study of obese adults found the substance effective at decreasing carbohydrate intake, enhancing satiety, and significantly aiding weight loss.

Supplementation: The recommended dosage is 50 to 100 mg about an hour or two before bedtime. *Note: If you take antidepressant medications or dietary supplements for depression, don't use 5-HTP without first checking with your doctor.*

NATURAL SEDATIVES AND CALMING AGENTS

There are a number of natural sedatives you can add to your supplement program that will help you sleep better, and supplements that will also help you calm down after a stressful day. Plants like passionflower and valerian root have the most research supporting them but other herbs can also be helpful.

Herbs That Can Help You Sleep

Acyanthopanax obovatus root is a special variety of ginseng that improves the quality of sleep.

Ashwagandha is a traditional Indian herb that acts as a sedative and induces a calming effect.

California poppy is useful in treating sleeplessness; it acts as a sedative.

Catnip isn't just for your kitty. It soothes the nerves, is relaxing, and great for the digestion. It can be used to make a sleep-promoting tea.

Chamomile soothes the nerves. German chamomile is the most effective. It promotes well-being and is good for the digestion. A cup of chamomile tea before bedtime is relaxing and soothing, and it's an excellent way to promote sleep. *Note: If you are allergic to plants such as ragweed, you shouldn't use chamomile.*

Hops are used as a traditional remedy for insomnia caused by anxiety. For best use of this herb, fill a sachet-size pillow with hops and place it near your pillow at night.

Juncus effuses leaf provides relief from worry and stress, and allows people to fall asleep more easily.

Passionflower is a sedative herb that prepares the brain and body for sleep. It eases anxiety-induced insomnia. It's very calming and relieves muscle spasms that can be painful and keep you awake. It is advisable not to drive for several hours after use, since it does induce drowsiness.

Pearlicium is a variety of pearl powder that calms the central nervous system and improves sleep quality.

Valerian root has a sedating and tranquilizing effect. It can lead to a restful sleep without morning sleepiness or other side effects or dangers of addiction. Studies have shown that valerian has extremely beneficial effects for people who are having difficulty falling asleep and also for irregular sleepers (particularly women).

Ziziphas jujaba leaf has been used for thousands of years to promote deeper, more restful sleep. It has also been found to induce sleep more quickly and to promote R.E.M.

Natural Sleep Aids

Coffea Cruda is a homeopathic remedy used to relieve insomnia, anxiety, fatigue, sleeplessness, and jittery restless feelings. It helps with insomnia whether it is right at bedtime, after midnight, or around 3 AM. Since Coffea Cruda is a homeopathic extract from coffee, the remedy also helps with problems that arise from overuse of coffee.

Ignatia is a homeopathic remedy that is helpful for restlessness and light sleep, along with emotional upset and depression from grief.

Melatonin is an antioxidant, immune system protector, sleep regulator, and cancer inhibitor; it also prevents jet lag. This hormone is produced by the pineal gland (a master gland located in the center of the brain); it's secreted mostly at night, peaking around 2 to 3 AM. Melatonin is present in virtually every cell of the body, promoting immune system integrity and normal circadian rhythms.

Melatonin production peaks in the early years of life and begins to decline around age thirty-five; it is almost negligible in people over the age of sixty. Nicknamed "the chemical expression of darkness," it is produced almost exclusively in a light-free environment. Blood levels of melatonin are up to ten times greater at night than during the day. This high concentration of nighttime melatonin led scientists to conclude that the production of this hormone signals the rest of the body that it's time to sleep. Indeed, melatonin supplements have been used for decades to treat sleep-related problems, such as insomnia, sleep apnea, and jet lag.

Though it is effective, any amount over 1.5 mg is recommended only as a last resort because it is a powerful hormone. If you are not melatonin-deficient and begin taking a larger amount, your body will curtail its own melatonin production. A slowdown in the production of any hormone can begin a chain reaction of chemistry imbalance and adverse symptoms. Ideally, it is best to increase melatonin levels naturally with exposure to bright sunlight in the daytime (along with full-spectrum fluorescent bulbs in winter) and absolute darkness at night. You can also use one of melatonin's precursors, 5-hydroxytryptophan (5-HTP) as a supplement (see page 110).

Supplementation: 1 to 1.5 mg.

Nux vomica If you find yourself waking up too early in the morning (like 3 AM) and unable to go back to sleep, the homeopathic remedy nux vomica may be helpful.

Rescue Remedy is a combination of Bach Flower Essences that is especially beneficial in traumatic situations, stress, emergencies, after getting bad news, before an exam or job interview—actually any stressful situations where you may suddenly lose balance mentally. Rescue Remedy has been used successfully on stressful days filled with impatience, tension, and pressure. It can help you relax, get focused, and calm down. Place two drops on your wrist and rub your wrists together before bedtime to help your body relax. It can be found at most health food stores.

White chestnut is a Bach Flower Essence that can help calm and quiet a chattering mind. Place several drops under your tongue at night. Again, it can be found at most health food stores.

FOODS AND SUBSTANCES THAT CAN KEEP YOU AWAKE AT NIGHT

Diet is an especially important consideration when you are experiencing sleeplessness or not getting refreshing sleep. Intolerance to certain foods can cause sleep problems, and it is essential to discover which foods are the culprits. In a study (*Pediatrics* 1985) of infants, sleeplessness was eliminated by removing cow's milk from the diet and then reproduced by its reintroduction. Also, eating too much, the consumption of caffeine or sweets, and the intake of drugs or alcohol are all important considerations when it comes to your sleep hygiene.

FOODS AND DRINKS TO AVOID

- Alcohol
- Additives and preservatives
- Coffee
- Chocolate candy, ice cream, or desserts
- Chocolate milk, hot chocolate, or cocoa
- Desserts and sweeteners
- Nonorganic foods containing pesticides
- Onions
- Rich sauces
- Spicy foods
- Soft drinks
- Tea (non-herbal)

Alcohol. As mentioned in Chapter 2, drinking alcohol can reduce your quality of sleep. In addition to causing the release of adrenaline, alcohol impairs the transport of tryptophan into the brain. It also disrupts serotonin levels because the brain is dependent upon tryptophan as a precursor for serotonin (an important neurotransmitter that initiates sleep). Also, if you're prone to low blood sugar, alcohol can contribute to nocturnal hypoglycemia (awakening in the night). In addition, alcohol and caffeinated beverages are dehydrating and somewhat irritating for the kidneys to process.

Antacids. Small amounts of aluminum are absorbed daily from air and water as well as from aluminum cooking utensils and some antiperspirants. But be especially aware of antacids, says James C. Penland, PhD, head researcher with the US Department of Agriculture. If you regularly take an antacid, especially a liquid, you should be conscious that many brands contain as much as 200 to 250 mg of aluminum per teaspoon. Dr. Penland suggests that if you take an antacid and find yourself waking up during the night, try giving it up for a few weeks to see if your sleep improves. It's best to give it up for other health reasons as well, since aluminum has adverse effects on health in general and has been associated with Alzheimer's.

Caffeine. In a world that values vigilance and productivity over rest and revitalization, caffeine has become, in dollar amounts, the second largest commodity (after oil) traded in the world. Some consumers require ever-greater jolts of caffeine. For example, a twenty-four-ounce coffee-bar cup of java can pack as much as 1,000 mg of caffeine; a typical cup of coffee is 100 mg. Caffeine has been associated with insomnia, restless legs syndrome, and nocturnal myoclonus (a neuromuscular disorder involving repeated contractions of one or more muscle groups, usually in the legs). Adenosine (a component of nucleic acids and energy-carrying molecules such as ATP) has long been known to promote sleep; its effects are blocked by caffeine. Just a few cups of coffee in the morning can interfere with your quality and quantity of sleep at night. Even the small amounts of caffeine in decaf coffee may be enough to affect some people who are very sensitive to stimulants. Coffee and other sources of caffeine such as tea (black and green, although green tea has only about one-third the caffeine of coffee), soda pop, chocolate, hot cocoa, and chocolate- and coffee-flavored ice cream should be avoided. Also, cold and cough medications often contain caffeine or caffeine-related substances.

CAFFEINE: THE NEMESIS OF THOSE COVETED ZZZS

The next time you're standing in line for that Mocha Latte Venti, consider this: Caffeine speeds up the action of many systems in your body. Within fifteen minutes of downing a cup of coffee, the adrenaline level in your bloodsteam rises, which triggers an increase in heart rate, breathing rate, urinary output, and production of stomach acids. Caffeine also prompts adrenal hormones to release sugar stored in the liver, which stimulates sugar cravings to replenish the stores. Caffeine promotes blood sugar swings, producing a quick high, followed by a letdown.

This is what you don't want to happen before you go to sleep. So you'd think that if you just drank coffee or tea in the morning, you'd be okay. But when some people drink coffee in the morning, it's still affecting them at night. Still, for most of us, the effects of caffeine wear off within about seven hours, so coffee in the morning will usually not interfere with sleep in the evening. Caffeine-containing beverages at lunch may or may not affect your sleep, but coffee, tea, chocolate, or cola in the evening is quite likely to keep you awake.

The best way to determine if the java you drink in the morning, iced tea at lunch, or hot cocoa at night is keeping you awake is to eliminate everything with caffeine and see if your sleep improves. Give it a few weeks and make note of any improvement.

Cigarettes and tobacco. While smoking may seem to have a calming effect, nicotine is actually a neurostimulant and can cause sleep problems.

Drugs and medications. There are more than three hundred drugs that interfere with normal sleep. Certain drugs can lead to insomnia, such as thyroid medication (also note that hypothyroidism can cause insomnia), oral contraceptives, beta-blockers, and marijuana. Even some over-the-counter drugs can cause abnormal sleep patterns. Check with your pharmacist or doctor about any medications you may be taking that might disrupt your sleep. If you're taking something that's known to cause sleep problems, ask your doctor if there is an alternative.

Food allergies and intolerances. Food sensitivities, intolerances, and allergies can significantly contribute to sleep disorders. Food-sensitive individuals often experience tension, restlessness, inattentiveness, and jitteriness during the day, as well as sleep disorders at night—including trouble getting to sleep, staying asleep, or getting up in the morning. In addition, tossing about all night or crying out during the night can be manifestations of food intolerances, as can nightmares. People who suffer from various food sensitivities are often irritable in the morning and sleepy in the afternoon, needing either a nap or a caffeinated drink to keep going.

Consuming foods we're intolerant of or allergic to can cause histamine (a substance produced in the body during an allergic reaction) to be released in the brain, affecting mood, thinking, and behavior; in some cases this can lead to sleep disorders. Common foods that cause reactions include dairy products, chocolate, sugar, wheat, shellfish, and corn. You could either get an allergy test or try an elimination diet, which means eliminating the foods noted above for six weeks and then adding them back one at a time to see if you react.

Food colorings and dyes can act as stimulants and contribute to insomnia. They have been associated with ADD and ADHD. Be aware that dyes and colorings are found in many products you might not expect—like packaged foods, breakfast cereal, soda pop, candy, gum, toothpaste, mouthwash, liquid antihistamine and other medications, even farm-raised salmon. Read labels and avoid anything that has added dyes or colorings.

AMERICA'S SUGAR LOAD

Ours is a generation of sugar babies: We've grown up on sugar with nearly every meal. Moreover, foods don't have to taste sweet to turn to sugar in the body. Bread, pasta, bagels, cereal, crackers, rolls, pizza, rice, corn, and potatoes—all turn to sugar, and some of these foods are eaten at nearly every meal in America. Then we wash it all down with a big glass of fruit juice, soda pop, a milk shake, or some wine. This high-carb soup all turns to sugar in the body and messes up our metabolism. It's no wonder our hormones are out of whack, we're overweight and insulin- and leptin-resistant, and we can't sleep well.

Monosodium glutamate (MSG) is often found in Chinese food; it causes a stimulant reaction in some people.

Sugars, sweeteners, and other refined carbohydrates all drain B vitamins. These foods also raise blood sugar levels, causing a burst

MENOPAUSE, INSOMNIA, AND SWEETS

Linda Ojeda, author of *Menopause Without Medicine,* says that after-dinner sweets, specialty coffees, and dinner wines, as comforting as they may seem, do not serve menopausal women well. If you are perimenopausal or you're already into menopause, you may have noticed that you aren't tolerating your favorite treats as well as you did a few years ago. The same coffee and chocolate at night that delighted you before may now keep you up until dawn staring at the ceiling or tossing and turning with nightmares, a racing heart, and hot flashes. Pay attention to foods that are no longer worth the momentary pleasure.

of energy that disturbs sleep. Eating sugar before bed often results in high blood sugar (hyperglycemia) for a short while, then—often after you go to sleep—your blood sugar drops to low levels (hypoglycemia); this is thought to contribute to restlessness, frequent awakenings, and nightmares. (Eating sugary, spicy, or exotic foods, drinking alcohol, or taking drugs before bedtime can also precipitate nightmares.) Probably the most important reason to avoid sugar and refined carbs is to reverse or prevent leptin and insulin resistance.

Tyramine-containing foods. Tyramine is an amino acid that increases the release of norepinephrine, which has a brain-stimulating effect and can keep you awake. Avoid bacon, cheese, chocolate, eggplant, ham, potatoes, sauerkraut, sugar, sausage, spinach, tomatoes, and wine, especially close to bedtime.

YOUR PRESCRIPTION FOR EATING WELL TO SLEEP AWAY THE POUNDS

- Follow a no-sugar diet.
- Include plenty of omega-3-rich foods, such as fish, leafy green vegetables, seeds, and nuts.
- Eat lots of brightly colored vegetables and low-sugar fruit.
- Avoid the foods that keep you awake and pack on the pounds.
- Include supplements that help you sleep and promote weight loss.

CHAPTER SIX)

Extra Help for Balancing Your Body Chemistry

If it seems you've tried everything, and you're still not achieving restorative sleep and slimming down, an out-of-balance endocrine system could be the culprit. This imbalance also may be contributing to a number of other health problems. Sleep is a physiological function that is controlled by hormones, which are released by endocrine system glands according to a natural cycle. A person who is struggling to lose weight and suspects that a lack of sleep is part of the reason for the difficulty can be experiencing a disruption in this natural cycle.

The endocrine system is a collection of glands and organs that produce and regulate hormones that control sleeping, waking, and appetite, along with many other bodily functions. The major glands of the endocrine system are the pituitary, hypothalamus, and pineal located in the brain, the thyroid and parathyroid in the neck, the thymus in the upper chest, the adrenals and pancreas in the upper abdomen, and the gonads, either ovaries or testes, in the lower abdomen. These glands regulate everything from when we fall asleep to when we reach our adult height.

The endocrine system is intricately involved in the sleep–wake cycle and weight management. For example, the pineal gland makes melatonin, which tells our body to sleep when it's dark and awaken when it's light. The pancreas produces insulin; if that production is off, we may not sleep through the night and may experience blood sugar imbalances, which affect our weight. The thyroid gland is involved in metabolism, and if its function is low, we may experience insomnia and weight gain. The hypothalamus regulates sleep and stimulates appetite and if it is out of whack, we may experience sleeplessness and a strong urge to overeat. The adrenals are responsible for adrenocorticotropin, adrenaline, cortisone, and cortisol levels. Some of these hormones regulate our sleep–wake cycle and fat deposits. If the adrenals are out of balance, we may wake up in the night, or we may have difficulty falling asleep when we turn the lights out. Known as the stress hormone, which can spike throughout the day when we're stressed out, cortisol is also responsible for fat deposits, especially on the abdomen. The amount of cortisol that is circulating in the body at any time is governed by complex interactions among the hypothalamus, pituitary gland, and adrenal glands. (This regulatory system is referred to as the hypothalamus-pituitary-adrenal axis, or HPA axis.) It is possible that sleep disturbances, including early-morning awakening, could be related to hyperactivity of the HPA axis. Indeed, hormone secretions have been shown to be imbalanced in patients with a dysfunctional HPA axis.

Sleep deprivation or disruption can have a significant impact on the endocrine system, which can have a major influence on sleep and weight gain. And thus the problem becomes magnified as sleep deprivation due to imbalanced hormones causes a worsening of endocrine function.

In the sections that follow, we'll look at specific glands—including the adrenals, hypothalamus, and thyroid—and what can be done to improve their health. The healthier the glands of your endocrine system, the better you'll sleep, and the faster your body will drop the weight you want to drop.

SUNLIGHT, SLEEP, AND THE ENDOCRINE SYSTEM

Have you noticed that you feel better and sleep better in summer or on vacation when you spend time outside? One of the most important factors in setting the natural rhythms of the sleep–wake cycle is exposure to natural sunlight. In fact, getting natural sunlight during the day often corrects sleeping problems. It may sound simple, but exposure to sunlight is fundamental to healthy sleep cycles. This is due to the production and suppression of melatonin—the sleep hormone. Melatonin levels normally rise at night and peak during sleep. Once you wake up, go outside, and receive natural sunlight exposure, melatonin levels are suppressed. This tells the body that it's morning and time to become alert.

When you avoid sunlight—if you have an office job, for instance, or purposely shun sunshine—and get only artificial light during the day, your melatonin levels may not be suppressed during the day. They can remain high, which tells the body that it may still be night. This may be one reason some people feel drowsy during the day, then can't sleep at night.

Get sunlight whenever possible to suppress daytime melatonin levels. And make sure your bedroom is dark at night to bring melatonin levels up. If you live in a climate where you can't get much natural sunlight, especially in winter, you can get full-spectrum lights. However, these bulbs are not a replacement for natural sunlight. You may need a winter vacation in a sunny climate.

STRESSED-OUT ADRENALS

At his lecture at the 2005 Complementary and Alternative Medicine Conference (CAMCON), sleep therapist Dr. Rubin Naiman said that 76 percent of Americans have a sleeping disorder at least a few days per week, contributing to our society's epidemic of daytime sleepiness, depression, and adrenal fatigue.

If you have struggled to find answers to your sleep problems, it could be that stressed-out adrenal glands are what's keeping you awake. This creates a vicious cycle of endless sleepless nights, fatigue, and added stress to already stressed adrenals. A number of doctors who deal with such issues estimate that 80 percent of Americans will suffer from some level of adrenal dysfunction at some time in their life, but most people will never know what it is. In fact, there isn't a lot of awareness of this condition even among those in the medical profession.

Almost all of us will admit we're stressed out many days of our lives. And for good reason! But all the stress, whether it's physical, emotional, mental, or environmental, is having a major impact on our adrenal glands. These glands respond to every kind of stress in the same way—they become more and more exhausted and dysfunctional. And dysfunctional adrenal glands have a major impact on our quality of sleep.

Scientists have found increased blood levels of stress hormones in people with chronic insomnia, suggesting that these individuals suffer from round-the-clock activation of the body's system for responding to stress. Hyperarousal of the adrenal glands can cause ongoing insomnia.

It appears that many people are experiencing sleep problems today because of stress leading to adrenal dysfunction. The stressors that people face in the twenty-first century are numerous and relentless. Long gone are the brief, alarm-phase reactions to acute stress. Modern people, instead of fighting for survival against

CORTISOL AND WEIGHT GAIN

Cortisol is a hormone produced in the adrenal cortex. It is important in the stress reaction and in regulating blood sugar and fat deposition. It's also responsible for energizing people in the morning or, when they're off cycle, for keeping them awake at night. People with low cortisol levels in the morning or afternoon will often try to bolster lagging energy by eating more food or drinking coffee. Consuming too much fast food, sweets, refined carbs such as white flour products, and caffeine will temporarily increase cortisol levels by driving the adrenals to produce hormones. (Alcohol also has this effect.) This causes weight gain, because even a temporary excess of cortisol causes fat to be deposited, especially around the midsection. This contributes to the spare tire or "swallowed beach ball" appearance. To correct this scenario of fatigue in the morning and afternoon with temporary bursts of cortisol due to quick-fix foods and drinks, it is very important to follow the healthy-diet suggestions in Correcting Adrenal Dysfunction (see page 127) and return your adrenal glands to normal function. In so doing, you can expect to see excess weight—especially belly fat—disappear, and to get more refreshing sleep at night.

predators, exposure to the elements, and starvation, are faced with stressors that seem never to go away such as bills, traffic, e-mails, career challenges, taxes, endless to-do lists, carpools for kids, eating on the run, poor diet, appointments, relationship issues, and money problems, to name just a few.

Abuse of the adrenal glands can cause dysfunction such as under- or overactivity. When overreacting or malfunctioning, the adrenals can pump out high levels of adrenal hormones in the evening or at bedtime, just when you should be winding down and getting ready

STRESSORS THAT CAN TRIGGER
ADRENAL DYSFUNCTION

- Anger
- Fear
- Worry
- Anxiety
- Guilt
- Too many carbohydrates
- Too little protein
- Severe allergies
- Stressful relationships
- Stressful job
- Insufficient sleep (both cause and effect)

- Chronic infections (such as flu and colds)
- Temperature extremes
- Light disruption (graveyard shift)
- Toxic exposure
- Chronic pain
- Chronic inflammation
- Surgery, trauma, injury
- Disease or illness
- Overwork

to sleep. Or they can start pumping out hormones in the middle of the night and wake you up; you may not be able to return to sleep.

In a normal cycle, cortisol output is highest first thing in the morning; it decreases from there, becoming the lowest around midnight. Both too-high and too-low levels of cortisol result in sleep disorders. For example, some people with stressed-out adrenals have high cortisol levels at bedtime or in the middle of the night. This imbalance interferes with sleep and produces a variety of "hyper" physical and mental symptoms. That's when you find yourself staring at the ceiling at 3 AM, mulling over the grocery list, the argument with your boss, and how you could have avoided the traffic ticket you got that week—all in rapid succession. You may feel energized and ready to get up and start the laundry or answer e-mails. But you know you'll pay a hefty price the next day for lack of sleep, so you lie there intent on drifting off again to slumberland . . . which doesn't

SYMPTOMS OF ADRENAL DYSFUNCTION

If your energy lags during the day, you often feel emotionally unbalanced, you sleep poorly or less than seven hours a night and don't feel rested when you awaken, you can't lose weight easily even when dieting, or you use caffeine or carbohydrates as pick-me-ups—you may have adrenal dysfunction. Following are some of the many symptoms associated with this disorder:

- Fatigue/lethargy
- Nervousness
- Depression
- Poor memory/concentration
- Low blood pressure
- PMS
- Low blood sugar (hypoglycemia)
- Dizziness/faintness
- Difficulty losing weight
- Inflammatory tendencies
- Dry or thin skin
- Poor resistance to illness
- Frequent infections
- Back/neck/shoulder/ muscle pain
- Difficulty getting up in the morning
- Decreased ability to handle stress
- Lapses in memory accuracy

- Weakness
- Irritability
- Digestive discomfort
- Light-headedness
- Insomnia
- Excessive hunger
- Craving for sweets
- Headaches
- Difficulty building muscle
- Low body temperature
- Limited perspiration
- Unexplained hair loss (head, underarms, legs)
- Muscle spasms
- Osteoporosis
- Craving for salt/ salty food
- Low sex drive
- Decreased productivity

happen, because your body is in a state of alert due to deranged hormonal activity.

For more in-depth information and help in determining if you have adrenal dysfunction, you may want to take the Adrenal Questionnaire in Dr. James. L. Wilson's book *Adrenal Fatigue: The 21st Century Stress Syndrome.*

CORRECTING ADRENAL DYSFUNCTION

A three-pronged approach is necessary to restore your adrenal glands to health and thereby resolve sleep and weight issues connected to adrenal dysfunction—lifestyle changes, dietary changes, and nutritional supplements.

Lifestyle changes involve stress reduction, relaxation, low-impact exercise, and reordering your life to remove some of the pressure. You may need to eliminate everything you can that's contributing to your stress, or rearrange your schedule to better manage your life. Many things cannot be removed or rearranged, though, including your job, family, and driving in traffic; therefore, it is vital to change how you view stressful situations and become more effective in dealing with them. Techniques for effectively responding to stress are found in Chapter 3.

Dietary changes are an important key to recovery. The best diet for adrenal dysfunction is one free of sugars and simple carbohydrates, rich in essential fatty acids and other good fats—both mono-unsaturated and saturated (yes, *saturated*; avoiding all saturated fats removes the type of fat used to make adrenal hormones, estrogen, and androgen)—as well as vegetables, low-sugar fruit, lean proteins, and fiber. Avoid sweets and simple and refined carbohydrates; these only compound blood sugar problems, which are associated with adrenal dysfunction and place further stress on the adrenal glands. (A number of doctors and nutritionists believe you will never totally

ADRENAL FUNCTION TESTS

With poor adrenal activity, blood pressure is usually low (105/60) on standing (postural hypotension) and then elevated (120 or 130/70 or 80) on reclining. (If you have too much aldosterone—which is an adrenal hormone that balances salt and water—your blood pressure will be high, and you may experience muscle pain and spasms.) This change from low to higher blood pressure when lying down may be why many people find it difficult to fall asleep. If this is true for you, you may want to lie in a semi-reclining position for the first fifteen or twenty minutes after going to bed.

A simple test based on blood pressure measurement can determine the likelihood of low adrenal function. Take your blood pressure sitting or lying down. Then, with the blood pressure cuff on, stand up quickly and immediately take your blood pressure again. In a normal person, the blood pressure should go up. In an adrenal-deficient person, it can go down (which is what contributes to light-headedness when standing up quickly from a reclining position). This test will not indicate adrenal dysfunction, such as releasing too much cortisol at night or a hyper state, where cortisol doesn't wind down. It's only helpful for hypoadrenia—low adrenal function.

You may also want to ask a health care professional about a saliva hormone test, which measures adrenal hormones in your saliva, rather than your blood. Saliva is more accurate than a blood test for adrenal hormones because it indicates amounts of hormones inside the cells where hormone reactions are taking place. It can also measure hormone levels at various times of the day and night, since you can place a saliva sample in a vial anytime. The only drawback is that you may need to search for a holistic doctor who uses these tests.

heal your adrenals and rebalance your HPA axis until you omit all sweets, refined carbohydrates, and alcohol. All of these turn rapidly to sugar in your bloodstream.)

There are a number of foods and substances that you should completely avoid to correct adrenal dysfunction. It may seem difficult, on a cold day, to order an herbal tea when everyone else is enjoying lattes or hot chocolate, but your well-rested, trim body will thank you. Take heed of the following tips.

Stay away from caffeine. Caffeine serves to increase the rate at which energy is consumed, thereby leading to further exhaustion of the adrenal glands. Sanford Bolton, PhD, from St. John's University in Jamaica, New York, found that habitual coffee drinkers had diminished adrenal function. Caffeine's action on stressed-out adrenal glands is like the inexcusable action of whipping an exhausted horse to make him run—the adrenals will pump out hormones so you feel temporarily better, but your glandular function will progressively become worse and you'll become more fatigued.

Caffeine is known as a metabolic disrupter. Perhaps the most frequently abused stimulants of all are coffee and soda. People who drink caffeine on a regular basis usually do so because they feel sleepy and fatigued in the morning—often because they have not had a good night's sleep in the first place. Drinking coffee to wake up creates an unhealthy cycle. The caffeine perks you up in the morning, but at the same time it puts stress on the whole endocrine system, which causes hormonal imbalances later on during the day. Then you feel tired in the afternoon and need something to pick you up. This can be particularly damaging over a long period of time. As a consequence, production of melatonin, cortisol, and other hormones is disrupted in the long term.

The best advice is to get off caffeine permanently. In his book *The New Detox Diet*, Elson M. Hass teaches people how to get off caffeine and why it's toxic to the nervous system. If you aren't sleeping well, you want to feed and heal your central nervous system, not stress it.

Don't use alcohol. Wine, beer, liquor—all forms of alcohol are very draining on the adrenal glands, since they turn to sugar very rapidly in the bloodstream.

Say no to MSG! MSG is a toxic substance that can cause sleep disorders and migraine headaches. It can also interfere with normal appetite regulation and make it almost impossible for people to lose weight. Read food labels carefully, because it's often included in grocery store products.

To improve adrenal health, here's what you *can* do to support these glands.

Eat meals at regular times. It's important to eat meals at regular times, as well as a small, healthy snack such as almonds or veggie sticks midmorning and midafternoon, if you suffer from adrenal fatigue. This will help keep cortisol levels more even throughout the day and maintain your energy.

Exercise elevates cortisol levels, so it's important to exercise regularly to improve depressed cortisol levels. It also helps balance irregular cortisol levels.

Don't exclude salt. We've all been told to avoid salt—but people with low adrenal function need it. Those with dysfunctional adrenals often tend to be salt losers, with a tendency to lose salt and retain potassium. You may retain fluids because your body is trying to hold on to salt. When adequate salt is consumed, the body will take what it needs and excrete the rest. Often, edema (the buildup of fluids) will disappear a few days after you add a little more salt to your diet. Adding Celtic or gray sea salt (which is rich in minerals, unrefined, and free of chemical additives) and sodium-rich foods such as kelp, dulse, olives, dill pickles, sauerkraut, and celery to your diet can be beneficial.

Salt is needed for heart action, to make hydrochloric acid in the stomach, and for the fluid around the cells. This extracellular fluid affects the proper function of muscles and cells. So go ahead—you can add a reasonable amount of salt to your food without guilt. Note: Plain table salt, which has additives, is not recommended. If you find that you need more sodium than potassium (which is in Celtic and gray sea salt), then choose kosher salt, plain sodium chloride without additives.

Supplements for Correcting Adrenal Function

Vitamin C is considered one of the most important nutrients in adrenal metabolism. The adrenal glands are one of the areas of the body where vitamin C concentrates. Vitamin C is quickly utilized in the body. Humans must ingest it because, unlike animals, we don't manufacture it in our bodies. Replacement is always necessary and extra vitamin C is needed when we're exposed to extensive activity, stress, illness, or oxidative processes. Long-term stress is thought to compromise the amount of stored vitamin C in the adrenal glands. Additionally, vitamin C is necessary for the synthesis of two important hormones, norepinephrine and epinephrine (adrenaline), which are produced during times of stress.

If you are experiencing a stressful situation, always increase your intake of vitamin C. For example, if you are going to be up late, have experienced an emotional crisis, are ill, have eaten junk food or food you are allergic to, have traveled across time zones, or have experienced any other stressful situation, increase your vitamin C supplementation.

Ascorbic acid (vitamin C) is typically synthesized from cane or beet sugar. It should be taken with bioflavonoids, which are essential for best utilization. The best ratio is two-to-one ascorbic acid to bioflavonoids. For example, if you are taking 1,000 mg of ascorbic acid, also take 500 mg of bioflavonoids. Often naturopathic physicians suggest a way to find the amount of vitamin C your body needs: Increase the ascorbic acid by increments of 500 mg, and bioflavonoids by 250 mg, until your stool becomes loose. Once you have achieved this level, reduce your ascorbic acid by 500 mg and your bioflavonoids by 250 mg or until your stool is no longer loose. The most common point for this to occur is between 2,000 mg and 4,000 mg of ascorbic acid and 1,000 to 2,000 mg of bioflavonoids. However, Dr. James Wilson, author of *Adrenal Fatigue,* says that he has known people who have required between 15,000 and 20,000 mg of vitamin C a day to reach this point. One word of caution: At amounts that high, it's best to be under a physician's care. When you cut back on your vitamin C/bioflavonoid regimen, do so gradually, in increments of 500/250 mg. A sudden drop can lead to symptoms of scurvy.

Vitamin B$_5$ (pantothenic acid) carries out its many functions in the body as part of the enzyme complex coenzyme A (CoA). CoA is involved in adrenal cortex function—it serves to increase production of glucocorticoids and other adrenal hormones. Research utilizing B$_5$ in laboratory animals shows that it enhances adrenal cortical function. Additionally, as part of CoA, B$_5$ is necessary for proper metabolism of carbohydrates and fats (leading to energy production) and the synthesis of the neurotransmitter acetylcholine. Vitamin B$_5$ is found in many foods, such as brewer's yeast, egg yolks, cheese, peanuts, fish, chicken, and numerous vegetables. It is also made in the intestines by the good bacterial flora. Despite the widespread availability of this vitamin, supplementation with B$_5$ is recommended for adrenal support. The recommended therapeutic dosage is 1,500 mg. It is best utilized when taken with the other B vitamins in a complex.

Magnesium acts like a spark plug for the adrenal glands. It is vital in the production of enzymes and energy needed for the adrenal hormone cascade and it will help you sleep well. Magnesium works with vitamins C and B_5 to improve the action of the adrenals. It's absorbed best after 8 PM and should be taken with an acid such as tomato or apple juice, a little fruit, or vitamin C powder in water. The recommended dosage is 400 mg; the best form is magnesium citrate in capsule or powder.

Licorice (*Glycyrrhiza glabra* and *G. uralensis*) helps reduce the amount of hydrocortisone broken down by the liver, thereby reducing the workload of the adrenal glands. Licorice has also been used to decrease symptoms of hypoglycemia, a common side effect of poor adrenal function. Commercial brands of licorice candy no longer contain real licorice; these products use aniseed and sugar, which taste similar but will not be helpful. Natural brands of licorice candy found in health food stores usually contain sweeteners, which should also be avoided. For adrenal support, only use real licorice in teas or supplements.

Long-term use of licorice containing more than 1 gram of glycyrrhizin (the amount in approximately 10 grams of licorice root) daily can cause increased blood pressure and water retention (edema). High doses of licorice and long-term use should be administered only under the care of a qualified health professional.

Adrenal cortical cell extracts are glandulars used to support and restore normal adrenal function. Not all holistic physicians recommend them. But some, such as Dr. James Wilson, find significant value in using them to treat adrenal dysfunction and accelerate recovery. Though a few companies do sell these extracts directly to the public, it is best to go through a health professional who can monitor your progress. (See Resources for recommended products.)

Analyzing the Results

When you combine a complete lifestyle change with diet changes and supplementation, it should take about three months to see significant improvements in your adrenal functioning, but some improvements may be noticeable in a few days. For some people, it can take up to two years for the adrenal glands to completely heal. Most people do recover when they incorporate the full program.

A STRESSED HYPOTHALAMUS

A hypothalamus gland that is not functioning properly can have a negative impact on sleep and weight loss. In a study published in *Cell Metabolism* (2005) involving mice and human cells, researchers traced the link between sleep debt and obesity to hypocretin and orexin, neuropeptides in the hypothalamus region of the brain that have a major impact on sleep and wakefulness. Brain cells have many times more nerve junctions that excite them than they have inhibitory contacts, making them easily excited and sensitive to stress. These specialized brain cells are particularly vulnerable to overstimulation and lack the ability of most other neurons to filter out signals from other regions of the brain that aren't meant for them. If these cells are overstimulated by environmental, physical, or mental/emotional stress in daily situations, they may encourage sustained arousal, generating sleeplessness and overeating. In this study, it was found that elevated hypocretin levels induced arousal, increased food intake, and fat gain. The authors conclude, "This circuitry may also be an underlying cause of insomnia and associated metabolic disturbances, including obesity."

Hypothalamus Support

Supporting adrenal function, as previously discussed, and thyroid function will help the hypothalamus. You may also benefit by taking hypothalamus extract (a glandular) combined with 10 to 40 mg of manganese.

LOW THYROID FUNCTION

When thyroid hormones are deficient, hypothyroidism manifests. Because energy control is pivotal to thyroid function, hypothyroid is a condition of reduced energy—you can feel tired and cold, grow mentally sluggish, become constipated, have less appetite but gain weight, find it difficult to lose weight, feel sleepy during the day, and experience insomnia.

Correcting Thyroid Problems

Rather than simply taking thyroid medication, it is very important to identify the underlying causes of poor thyroid health. You may need to take medication until you have sufficiently restored healthy thyroid function. But simply taking thyroid hormone replacement drugs for a lifetime does not feed the thyroid or correct its dysfunction. Rather, it bypasses the thyroid. A high percentage of people with hypothyroidism also experience osteoporosis. This is no doubt due to the fact that the thyroid makes a hormone called calcitonin that facilitates absorption of calcium. Thyroid medication can also contribute to insomnia and other sleep problems.

Here are some things you *can* do to nourish your thyroid.

Eat only healthy fats and oils. Virgin coconut oil, unrefined extra-virgin olive oil, and fish oil are the healthiest choices. Virgin coconut oil has helped many people restore healthy thyroid function. Polyunsaturated oils—including sunflower, safflower, corn, and soy—are not recommended. Soy oil is a goitrogen, which means it blocks iodine absorption; iodine is a very important nutrient for thyroid health. Be aware that most commercial salad dressings and mayonnaise contain soybean oil. Perhaps the single most important dietary change you can make is to replace polyunsaturated vegetable oils with coconut and olive oils in food preparation.

Consume plenty of iodine-rich foods. Iodine is most abundant in sea vegetables, cranberries, fish, and eggs. Season foods with dulse or kelp powder in place of regular table salt. Use Celtic or gray sea salt whenever possible; it's loaded with minerals, including iodine. Eat fish regularly, especially the smaller cold-water fish such as salmon (avoid farm-raised), mackerel, sole, sardines, and snapper. Avoid larger species such as tuna and swordfish; they tend to be higher in mercury, which interferes with thyroid function.

Take vitamin and mineral supplements and cod-liver oil. A number of nutrients have been shown to contribute to thyroid health, including zinc, selenium, manganese, chromium, B vitamins, and vitamins C, E, and A. The thyroid gland requires very high levels of vitamin A. Individuals with hypothyroidism have been shown to have an impaired ability to convert beta-carotene to vitamin A, so take care to include vitamin A supplements. Cod-liver oil is a very good source of natural vitamin A. Choose cod-liver oil from cod caught in Icelandic or Norwegian waters, where fish are less likely to have high mercury levels.

Avoid goitrogens. Foods known as goitrogens can block iodine from being absorbed by the thyroid gland. These include turnips, cabbage, broccoli, cauliflower, Brussels sprouts, raw spinach (cooked is okay), mustard, pine nuts, millet, peanuts, almonds, and soybeans. Until your thyroid health is restored, you may want to avoid these foods completely, or eat them very sparingly. Peanuts and soybeans are quite prevalent in the American diet. Soy shows up often in many commercially made salad dressings, mayonnaise, and packaged foods containing textured vegetable protein (soy), such as veggie burgers, energy bars, snack foods, and baked goods. Soy milk and soy ice cream are commonly used as alternatives to dairy. Choose only traditional fermented soy foods such as tofu, tempeh, and soy sauce, and eat those sparingly.

CHAPTER SEVEN

Solutions for Insomnia and Other Sleep Disorders

An old Chinese proverb states, *Only when you cannot sleep do you know how long the night is.* When you watch a baby drift effortlessly to sleep or observe your dog go from sixty to zero in a matter of seconds, you may feel a twinge of envy. If so, then you are probably no stranger to the challenges of falling asleep and staying asleep. Millions of people suffer from insomnia, and most of us will experience it at some point in our lives. There is nothing like staring at a darkened ceiling in the middle of the night to make you wish you could just circle the carpet a couple of times and then slumber like a contented pooch!

If you're not getting enough sleep each night, it's important to get to the bottom of what's keeping you awake. Perhaps there's something that's getting between you and a good night's sleep. Chapter 3 looked at an overactive mind, stress, and an inability to relax and let go. In Chapter 6 we looked at an imbalanced endocrine system and how to restore it. In this chapter, we'll look at insomnia and a number of other contributors to poor sleep such as nocturnal hypoglycemia, and various sleep disorders like restless legs syndrome and sleep apnea.

SLEEPLESS IN AMERICA

From time to time, almost all of us have experienced a sleepless night or two. But for an ever-growing number of people, sleeplessness is becoming a common occurrence. Close to 40 percent of the US population over the age of fifteen report they've experienced insomnia at least occasionally. A poll sponsored by the National Sleep Foundation found that 74 percent of respondents experienced at least one symptom of a sleep disorder a few nights a week; only 30 percent of adults reported getting eight or more hours of sleep on weeknights.

Insomnia affects about 40 percent of women and 30 percent of men in the United States. Women often have difficulty sleeping during periods of biological change when hormone levels rise and fall, such as menstruation, pregnancy, and menopause. Insomnia has also been found to be more frequent among shift workers and older adults.

For the more than seventy million Americans suffering from insomnia, sleep apnea, or other sleep disorders, functioning on little sleep is the norm rather than the exception. Such patterns can lead to serious sleep deficits, weight gain, and a host of health problems such as cancer, diabetes, heart disease, and obesity.

If you've experienced insomnia, you can no doubt rattle off a sizable list of symptoms you've experienced following a sleepless night—irritability, difficulty with concentration and memory, fatigue, erratic emotions, and increased hunger, just to name a few. Prolonged insomnia can leave you with decreased immune function and depression, and often has a negative impact on your relationships with other people, especially those with whom you live. Worse yet, frequent insomnia can set you up to fear another sleepless night, a phenomenon known as psychophysiological insomnia. That anxiety alone can keep you from falling asleep; if you awaken in the night, it can trigger a stress hormone release that can keep you awake till dawn. (Chapter 3 will help you deal with turning that scenario around.)

Not all sleeplessness is categorized as insomnia, but for at least seventy million people this sleep disorder is all too familiar.

WHAT IS INSOMNIA?

If you have trouble sleeping from time to time, it's not unusual. But if you fail to get enough sleep or satisfying sleep on a regular basis, you may have insomnia. Insomnia is defined as the inability to fall asleep or remain asleep. People who suffer from it may have trouble drifting off to sleep, may wake up frequently during the night, or may have difficulty returning to sleep once they awaken. Or they may wake up too early in the morning. In addition, they may experience daytime sleepiness, irritability, increased hunger, or difficulty concentrating.

Insomnia is not defined by the number of hours you sleep every night, because the amount of sleep we need varies. While most of us need between seven and nine hours each night, some people do well with less, and some need more. Rather, it is defined by the quality of the sleep and whether or not you feel refreshed and restored upon rising.

Insomnia can cause problems during the day, such as drowsiness, fatigue, excess hunger, difficulty concentrating, accidents, and irritability. A person with insomnia may also have another sleep disorder such as sleep apnea, narcolepsy, or restless legs syndrome. But solutions do exist for sleep issues, and when you get to the root of the causes, you should be drifting off to slumberland like a healthy baby and controlling your appetite far better than before.

TYPES OF INSOMNIA

Primary insomnia involves difficulty sleeping that is not related to other health conditions or medications.

Secondary insomnia involves sleep problems that occur because of a medical condition—for example, depression, hypothyroidism, fibromyalgia, heartburn, or cancer—or side effects of pharmaceutical drugs or other substances, such as alcohol or caffeine.

Some types of insomnia can vary in duration.

Acute insomnia is short-term, lasting from one night to a few weeks; often it is triggered by a significant or stressful event; by environmental factors, like temperature or noise; or by emotional or physical distress or disruptions in the sleep cycle, such as from jet lag or daylight saving time changes.

Intermittent insomnia occurs on and off in people who temporarily experience stress, noise, extreme temperature changes, schedule changes such as jet lag, and medical issue side effects.

Chronic insomnia is defined as having insomnia at least three nights a week for a month or longer. It may be the result of depression, persistent stress, chronic pain, or physical dysfunction such as adrenal fatigue, hypoglycemia, or low thyroid.

Psychophysiological insomnia occurs when you worry about whether or not you'll be able to fall asleep or stay asleep, which triggers insomnia.

WHAT YOU CAN DO TO CORRECT INSOMNIA

A good portion of this book is dedicated to helping you get a good night's sleep. Starting with Chapter 2, we offer scores of tips to help you experience a restful night of refreshing sleep. Chapter 3 offers tools to help you calm your mind and emotions, reduce stress, and relax so you can drift off to sleep easily. In Chapter 4, you discovered that exercise, the third step in our weight loss program, is as vitally important to a good night's sleep as it is for weight loss. Diet, which we discuss in Chapter 5, is also crucial to sleeping well. The low-sugar diet we present is as important to weight loss as it is for good sleep because sugar can pack on the pounds and keep you awake half the night. Balancing your biochemistry is the topic of Chapter 6, and may be your answer to solving long-standing sleep problems.

HELPFUL REMEDIES FOR SLEEPLESSNESS

Here are some quick-fix action steps you can take when you find yourself awake in the middle of the night.

Eat a little turkey or a protein snack if your blood sugar is low. Your liver may be lacking the glycogen reserves needed to keep blood glucose levels high enough during the night for restful sleep. If you are hypoglycemic, your blood sugar may fall so low that it wakes you up. (This can contribute to nightmares, fitful sleep, and anxiety attacks.) If this happens, get up and eat some turkey or another protein-rich snack. Turkey contains tryptophan, a major building block for making serotonin, a neurotransmitter, which sends messages between nerve cells and produces feelings of sleepiness. It will also help to stabilize your blood sugar. (Do not eat anything sweet; this will raise your blood sugar temporarily, and then drop it lower still, which could cause you to awaken.) Other foods, besides turkey, that contain a notable amount of tryptophan are cottage cheese, yogurt, chicken, almonds, cashews, and tuna. (Be careful of tuna because of mercury contamination.)

Take several deep breaths. Deep breathing is a reliable intervention when you wake up in the middle of the night. Take a slow deep breath, counting to four or five, hold it for a count of two, and then slowly release the air for a count of four or five. Do this several times until you fall back to sleep.

Take adrenal support supplements. These supplements can be helpful if your adrenal glands are stressed. (See Resources.)

Take a Calms Forté tablet. Calms Forté by Hyland's is a natural sleep aid that is a relaxant. Check your local health food store.

Take magnesium citrate and calcium citrate. A deficiency of calcium or magnesium can cause you to wake up in the night and not be able to return to sleep. It may be that you are particularly magnesium-deficient; many people are. A magnesium citrate powder mixed in water may help. *Check with your doctor before taking if you have heart or kidney problems.*

Take a B-complex vitamin with vitamin C and bioflavonoids. B vitamins are important for your nervous system and help you relax. Vitamin C and bioflavonoids are helpful for the adrenal glands.

Sniff lavender oil. Lavender has long been used for calming tension and anxiety. There are lavender oil inhalers that can be helpful.

Put a drop or two of Rescue Remedy on each wrist and rub them together. Rescue Remedy is a Bach Flower Essence that is helpful for tension, trauma, or anxiety. It is especially helpful to the body after a long day of travel. It's found at most health food stores.

Try white chestnut Bach Flower Essence to calm a chattering mind.

Put on a sleep tape. There are audio programs that offer guided sessions to help you manage anxiety and quiet your mind. Some of them have soothing music, even heartbeats, that put you into a meditative, relaxed state. Put on your earphones so you don't awaken anyone else in the house, lie back, and drift off.

BALANCE BRAIN CHEMISTRY AND SLEEP WELL AGAIN

Neurotransmitters (brain chemicals) play a large part in getting a good night's sleep. In fact, there's an interesting connection between brain chemicals and certain conditions that cause sleepless nights, as well as carbohydrate cravings and an inability to lose weight. They can all go hand in hand.

Neurotransmitters fall into two categories: excitatory (stimulating) and inhibitory (calming). A good sleep cycle depends on a very delicate balance of the two. First, you must have adequate levels of the calming neurotransmitter serotonin to synthesize enough melatonin for successful sleep. But a good night's sleep takes much more than that. The excitatory neurotransmitter norepinephrine must be optimal during the daytime and this level must fall by evening for sleep to ensue.

There are many signs of low serotonin levels such as carbohydrate cravings, exaggerated responses to stress, and a compromised immune system. If norepinephrine is not at optimal levels, then lack of motivation, focus, and poor energy can occur.

Testing neurotransmitter values through a scientific lab test is the only way to discover your unique neurotransmitter levels and determine where there may be imbalances. (And it's relatively inexpensive! See the Sleep Quiz on page 145 for more information.) Utilizing this analysis to create your customized Brain Wellness Program can make a significant difference in your sleep patterns, carb cravings, and weight loss.

We have worked with many people who have been tested and were found to have significant neurotransmitter imbalances. Working with amino acids targeted for individual needs, we've seen great improvement in sleep, carb cravings, and weight loss.

NEUROTRANSMITTERS

Serotonin is the master neurotransmitter. It is responsible for keeping a balance between excitatory and inhibitory neurotransmitters. When it's off balance, symptoms can arise, such as depression, anxiety, worry, obsessive thoughts and behaviors, carbohydrate cravings, PMS, difficulty controlling pain, and sleep disturbances. Or there may simply be lethargy (lack of energy and motivation). Serotonin is an inhibitory neurotransmitter, which means it doesn't stimulate the brain. Adequate amounts of serotonin are necessary for a stable mood and to balance any excessive excitatory (stimulating) neurotransmitters in the brain. Using stimulant medications or caffeine daily can cause a depletion of serotonin over time.

Epinephrine (also known as adrenaline) is an excitatory neurotransmitter that is indicative of stress. Long-term stress or insomnia can cause epinephrine levels to be depleted (low).

PEA, or phenylethylamine, is a neurotransmitter chemical in the brain that causes you to fall madly in love with someone. It is a natural form of amphetamine that floods the regions of the brain involved in sexual excitement. It also plays a role in attention, depression, and energy level. Elevated levels of PEA can cause

SLEEP QUIZ

1) **Do you have trouble falling asleep?**
   yes no
2) **Do you have trouble staying asleep?**
   yes no
3) **When you wake up, do you still feel tired?**
   yes no
4) **Do you have carbohydrate cravings?**
   yes no

If you answered yes to any of these questions, you may have a brain chemistry imbalance. You can determine if you do have an imbalance by taking a urinalysis test. The results will help determine exactly which amino acids can help you balance your brain chemistry.

anxiety and insomnia. Low levels often cause lethargy and a lack of focus. PEA may be at a level of 250–300 in the morning but it will frequently rise during the day while working up to 2,000 or more. It decreases as the day continues so that we can have an appropriate sleep cycle. When it remains high, sleep can be impaired.

Histamine is an excitatory neurotransmitter. It also plays a role in response to allergies and inflammation. High levels of histamine can cause agitation, irritability, and sleep cycle disturbances. Low levels of histamine are associated with feeling tired. Histamine also promotes the excretion of epinephrine and norepinephrine.

GETTING AT THE ROOTS OF INSOMNIA

If your sleep problems are persistent, you may need to do some detective work to get to the root of your problem. Read the information that follows and work on changing your health at the core level.

If you frequently awaken between 3 and 5 AM, consider the possibility of adrenal fatigue or dysfunction. Waking throughout the night can be adrenal-related. Dysfunctional adrenal glands have a major impact on your quality and quantity of sleep. Scientists have found increased blood levels of stress hormones in people with chronic insomnia, suggesting that these individuals suffer from round-the-clock activation of the body's system for responding to stress. This hyperarousal of the adrenal glands can cause ongoing insomnia.

The adrenal glands are responsible for releasing cortisol at appropriate times such as morning to arouse us naturally from sleep. Cortisol production should wind down in the evening and stay low through the night so we can sleep. But if the adrenal glands are out of balance or aroused due to stress, cortisol levels can remain high and keep us awake. If you've experienced stress of any kind— whether it's physical (such as trauma, illness, surgery, or injury), emotional or mental (such as divorce, the death of a loved one) or job or relationship problems, or environmental (such as exposure to chemicals or extreme temperatures)—your adrenal glands may be stressed out and dysfunctional as a result. Read Chapter 6 for more information and take the appropriate steps to heal your adrenal glands.

Cleanse your liver; a toxic or congested liver can keep you awake or cause you to awaken around 3 AM. According to Chinese medicine, chronic sleep disorders are often caused by yin–yang imbalance resulting from a weak liver, spleen, heart, or kidneys. Chinese medicine says the liver filters all our blood through the night, especially between 1 and 3 AM. A weak, toxic, or congested liver has to struggle during the night, and this can be one reason we awaken between 1 and 3 AM. Poor-quality sleep may result. Your sleep, weight loss program, and overall health may greatly benefit if you complete a liver-cleanse program.

Also, aging affects quality of sleep. Research indicates that around age forty, sleep patterns begin to change, resulting in more nocturnal awakenings. But if you are diligent about cleansing your colon, liver, gallbladder, and kidneys and rejuvenating your entire body, you can minimize these effects and sleep well into your golden years.

Improve digestion. Odd as it may seem, poor digestion will affect your sleep, not only because you may have uncomfortable indigestion that keeps you awake, but also because you may not be breaking down proteins and absorbing minerals. As you saw in Chapter 5, both amino acids and various minerals are very important to sleeping well. Hydrochloric acid and the enzyme pepsin are necessary for protein digestion and mineral absorption. If these digestive secretions are inhibited, proper protein digestion and mineral absorption will not occur. Stress can have a major impact on digestion because if you are in a stressed state, blood is shunted away from the digestive tract in favor of the skeletal muscles and brain. That's why regularly achieving a relaxed state, especially when you eat, and learning to calm your mind and body are so important to improving digestion. (See Chapter 3 for tips on quieting your mind.) You may find that taking digestive aids such as betaine HCl, pepsin, and digestive enzymes may be beneficial. Chiropractic care can also be very helpful in improving digestion.

Spinal structure imbalances should be corrected. Traditional chiropractic care can help with insomnia. It can help those with spasms, pain, and joint dysfunctions of the neck and back. The brain stem is involved in actions such as walking, sleeping, arousal, and lying down and can be affected by a misaligned skull or upper cervical vertebra. If any of these areas are out of alignment, you can experience insomnia.

Have your hormones checked, especially if you are menopausal or perimenopausal. Hormonal changes, and in particular low estrogen levels, can cause insomnia. (The type of hormones you take can be very important to your overall health. We recommend natural hormones. You may benefit by seeing a holistic physician or naturopathic doctor.)

Have your iron level tested. Iron-deficient women tend to have more problems sleeping. If your blood is iron-poor, you may need to include a little red meat in your diet once or twice a week along with a vitamin-C-rich food such as tomatoes or broccoli to maximize your iron absorption. Eat lots of leafy greens, as well. If the situation persists, see your doctor. (It is not recommended that you take iron supplements other than the small amount that may be in a multivitamin; these have been linked to cancer.)

Prevent sinus pain and sinus headaches. Sinus problems can keep you awake even when you're exhausted. A number of scientific studies have found that an herbal remedy known as Sinupret is very effective for symptomatic relief of sinus problems. It thins the mucus that clogs up the sinuses and lungs, allowing it to drain properly and promoting normal mucus flow. It also has anti-inflammatory activity, making it helpful for asthma and allergies. And its antiviral activity makes it helpful for colds and flu. (See Resources.)

Address hypothyroid issues. Low thyroid function can cause insomnia—and so can thyroid medication. It is important to feed the thyroid and improve its health, rather than simply bypassing it with thyroid medication. (Never stop taking such medication abruptly, but work with your doctor to wean yourself off it as you improve your thyroid health.) Follow the suggestions in Chapter 6 for improving thyroid health. Also, our book *The Coconut Diet* has an entire chapter devoted to achieving thyroid health, along with a thyroid health quiz.

THE PROS AND CONS OF SLEEPING PILLS

Since learning about how important it is to get a good night's sleep, you may be tempted to get some sleeping pills today and start sleeping. But it's important to know the pros and cons first. If you can't sleep night after night, it's far better to take a sleeping pill than stay awake for hours. The Mayo Clinic says sleeping pills help when stress, travel, or other disruptions keep you awake. But if you have chronic insomnia, a better approach is to remove the cause—most often, by changing your lifestyle. Sleeping pills can be addictive—if not physically, then at least psychologically. And they're not without side effects.

Thomas Roth, MD, director of the Sleep Disorders and Research Center at Henry Ford Health System in Detroit, says, "You want to use them [sleeping pills] in conjunction with good sleep practices, good behavioral therapies, and treating accompanying conditions. That means, among other things, practicing 'good sleep hygiene.'" It's important to get to the root of the problem and find out why you're not sleeping. Insomnia, defined as difficulty falling and/or staying asleep, or waking up too early, is usually the symptom of an underlying issue. (Chapter 6 and this chapter are devoted to helping you discover why you can't sleep well and helping you correct the underlying issues.)

Studies have also found that cognitive behavioral therapy (teaching people how to manage their thinking and behavior) can be a very effective treatment for insomnia, making it easier to fall asleep more quickly and stay asleep longer. Research shows that medications aren't as effective in the long term as behavioral treatment of insomnia. Changing behavior can have a greater impact and longer duration of effectiveness.

Still, while you're digging for the root of your sleepless nights and working on sleep interventions, a sleeping pill might make the difference between snoozing and having very little sleep night after night.

The pros. Nonbenzodiazepine hypnotic medications (Rozerem, Ambien, and Lunesta) are the newest class of sleeping pills. They bind to a specific benzodiazepine receptor in the brain, called omega-1, thereby inducing sleep. They may be less likely than benzodiazepine medications to disrupt natural rapid-eye-movement (REM) sleep rhythm patterns. Disruption of REM sleep may make sleep less restful. These medications are metabolized quickly, which helps reduce the risk of side effects the next day. They're mainly intended for short-term or intermittent use, and they're available by prescription only.

The older classes of sleep medications—benzodiazepines such as Valium and Xanax—alter sleep. They tend to decrease the amount of time spent in Stages 3 and 4 sleep (the deepest, most restful stages), and people often complain of hangover effects. Nonbenzodiazepine hypnotics, on the other hand, have a relatively short half-life, so people don't tend to wake up groggy the next day. They have little effect on sleep stages, allowing deep sleep. And they are less likely than other sleeping pills to cause addiction, withdrawal symptoms, or buildup of tolerance (a condition in which you require more and more drug to have the same effect).

Most over-the-counter sleep aids are antihistamines. This means they're sedating and can cause some drowsiness the next day. They're safe enough to be sold without a prescription, but be aware that if you're taking other drugs that have similar effects, such as cold or allergy medications, you could take too much.

The cons. Common side effects of nonbenzodiazepine hypnotics include drowsiness and dizziness, possibly impairing coordination, balance, and/or mental alertness. These drugs must be used with caution in individuals with a history of drug abuse or dependence. Ambien, Lunesta, and Rozerem work very quickly and should only be taken just before going to bed.

Ambien may cause dry mouth, diarrhea, dizziness, or prolonged drowsiness. It may not be safe for people who have a history of depression, liver or kidney disease, or respiratory conditions. It has been associated with memory loss, sleep-walking, and blackouts. It should be used mainly to help people fall asleep. Overuse is possible for people experiencing anxiety.

Rozerem should not be used if there is severe hepatic impairment or in combination with Luvox. It has been associated with decreased testosterone levels and increased prolactin levels. It should not be taken with or immediately after a high-fat meal and caution should be used when consuming alcohol. The most common adverse side effects are somnolence (daytime drowsiness), dizziness, and fatigue. It is indicated only for sleep-onset difficulties.

Lunesta may cause an unpleasant taste in the mouth, rash, nausea, vomiting, dizziness, headache, depression, swelling, reduced interest in sex, or chest pain. It may not be safe for pregnant women and people who have a history of drug or alcohol abuse, depression, lung disease, or a condition that affects metabolism. It is used mainly to help people stay asleep. Stopping the drug abruptly may cause withdrawal symptoms.

Antihistamines work against the central nervous system's chemical histamine and can be quite sedating. Sedation, however, isn't the same as good sleep, according to sleep specialist Karl Doghramji, and the sleep quality may be poor. Among the more serious side effects for people with neuromuscular disorders is that these medications tend to dry up respiratory secretions, making mucus harder to cough up and more likely to plug bronchioles (breathing tubes) in the lungs.

SLEEP DISORDERS AND WHAT
YOU CAN DO ABOUT THEM

You may not be getting enough restful sleep because of a sleep disorder other than insomnia. The International Classification of Sleep Disorders lists more than eighty types. Below are a number of those most often experienced and tips for overcoming these problems.

NOCTURNAL HYPOGLYCEMIA

A large percentage of people in the United States suffer from defective glucose metabolism, either as low blood sugar (hypoglycemia)

HYPOGLYCEMIA (LOW BLOOD SUGAR) SYMPTOMS

- Craving for sweets
- Irritability if meals are missed
- Tiredness or weakness if meals are missed
- Dizziness when standing suddenly
- Frequent headaches
- Poor memory (forgetfulness or lack of concentration)
- Fatigue after eating
- Heart palpitations
- Occasional shakiness
- Afternoon fatigue
- Occasional blurred vision
- Depression or mood swings
- Overweight
- Anxiety or nervousness

or high blood sugar (diabetes)—largely due to our Western lifestyle, which encourages overeating sugar and other refined carbohydrates and results in imbalanced hormones.

Low nighttime blood glucose, known as nocturnal hypoglycemia, is one cause of frequent or early awakening. Symptoms may include sweating, anxiety, hunger, tremors, or a sinking feeling. When there is a drop in your blood glucose level, it causes the release of hormones that regulate glucose, such as adrenaline, glucagon, cortisol, and growth hormone. These compounds send a message to the brain that it's time to eat—and then you're awake. Severe episodes can cause convulsions and coma and have been implicated as a precipitating factor in cardiac arrhythmias resulting in sudden death—known as the "dead-in-bed syndrome."

Managing Blood Sugar May Work Better Than Counting Sheep

To attain quality sleep and facilitate weight loss, it's very important to maintain balanced blood sugar levels at all times, especially during the night. This enables the body to dip into fat reserves while you are sleeping, an essential dynamic for healthy weight loss. This also enables the body to clear out toxins and make much-needed repairs to keep the body healthy and trim.

You may experience low blood sugar in the wee hours and not sleep soundly through the night because of nocturnal hypoglycemia. Imbalanced blood sugar levels can be driven by emotional and physical stress. When blood sugar is not balanced at bedtime or during the night, not only will you not sleep well, but you won't burn fat as efficiently, either. You may experience either elevated blood sugar or low blood sugar at bedtime. More people seem to experience elevated blood sugar because it doesn't take much to spike up those numbers. Ron Rosedale, MD, notes that one saltine cracker can take blood sugar higher than 100, and in many people it can take blood sugar over 150. Think what happens when you eat a bowl of sugary cereal flakes, a bagel, or a dish of ice cream!

If you have elevated blood sugar levels prior to going to bed, this can cause the body to feel like it's overworking when it should be relaxing. In such instances, you may be tired, even exhausted, but a racing feeling in your body will prevent you from relaxing and drifting off to slumberland. Your mind may take off with continual chatter. Your heart may race or skip a beat. Your energy will feel uncomfortable—unlike the energy you experience after a good night's sleep. In this state, you may begin to process the day's events as soon as your head hits the pillow. This generates stress responses, releasing adrenaline and cortisol. These stress hormones interfere with falling asleep, staying asleep, and sleeping deeply. Then you become anxious about not going to sleep, and the problem accelerates as your body pumps out more stress hormones.

Compounding the issue, elevated cortisol at bedtime depresses leptin function, which should be active during the night. (Remember, leptin is the hormone that curbs appetite.) By the time leptin gets going in the early-morning hours, it blunts cortisol release, just when it should be increasing; hence you wake up tired. Cortisol is meant to wake up your cells and get them ready for the day. (If this is you and your doctor orders a saliva test to measure adrenal function, your morning cortisol reading will be quite low.)

This hormonal imbalance can lead to a variety of symptoms, from waking up hungry in the night to nightmares, excess sweating, and headaches during sleep or upon waking. And rather than awakening energized and refreshed, you may drag out of bed feeling tired and dull, your head heavy and your mood irritable. You may end up grumpy half the morning. You may not remember things you need to do, and your brain may feel foggy and disconnected. You may have to get a cup of coffee or a caffeinated soda just to get started. You may also wake up hypoglycemic and need to eat something fairly quickly.

If you tend toward low blood sugar at bedtime, you will be apt to eat too much before going to bed. You may specifically crave sweets such as ice cream, cookies, or candy, or refined carbs like crackers, bread, or cereal. Such snacks can greatly interfere with fat burning during the night and leave you with elevated blood sugar that can eventually drop lower than when you started, causing you to wake up in the middle of the night.

Whether you have elevated blood sugar or low blood sugar at bedtime, it's a sign that overall fuel regulation is out of balance. Since sleep is the longest time for most of us to go without food, it serves as a good test of blood sugar balance, hormone balance, and liver fitness. If your blood sugar is out of balance, it is essential to bring it into equilibrium. It's also essential to balance your appetite-regulating hormones leptin, ghrelin, insulin, cortisol, and adrenaline so they can work together. You'll have an indication that healthy blood sugar, hormonal balance, and liver health are being restored when you sleep well through the night and wake up energized and refreshed in the morning without any need for caffeine or other stimulants to get going. Your appetite will be under control and you'll be able to make healthy food choices. And you'll experience optimum fat cell metabolism, meaning that weight loss and maintenance won't require as great an effort as before.

Dietary change, good sleep hygiene, and stress management are keys to accomplish this biochemical balance. And liver cleansing may be called for to achieve optimum liver health. Dr. Ron Rosedale says that simply taking drugs to artificially raise insulin and/or leptin will not correct the problems in orchestration of hormonal signals any more than playing a tuba louder will fix mistakes in written music. (That's not to say that you should discontinue any medication without a doctor's advice.) However, a strategic diet that emphasizes good fats and avoids blood sugar spikes—coupled with specific supplements to enhance insulin and leptin sensitivity by resensitizing your cells' ability to hear hormonal messages correctly, and managing your stress—will allow your life to be the symphony it was meant to be.

Correcting Nocturnal Hypoglycemia

If you suffer from nocturnal hypoglycemia, omit all refined and high-glycemic carbohydrates from your diet. (See Chapter 5 for more dietary tips.) Some people are so sensitive to sugars that even a small amount of sweetener can set off a hypoglycemic (low blood sugar) reaction. To help prevent nighttime low blood sugar, eat an evening snack that is high in fiber such as oatmeal or vegetables with hummus, or a small snack rich in tryptophan, such as a slice of turkey or a few almonds. Beyond these temporary quick fixes, it is important to learn how to manage your blood sugar, keeping it stable on an ongoing basis. See Chapters 5 and 6. And it is equally as important to learn to manage stress; see Chapter 3.

SLEEP-DISORDERED BREATHING:
SLEEP APNEA AND SNORING

Obstructive sleep apnea (OSA), or the early stages of development of a sleep apnea condition such as loud snoring, is a common sleep disorder characterized by brief interruptions of breathing during sleep. According to the National Institutes of Health, approximately twelve million Americans suffer from obstructive sleep apnea (OSA).

People who have OSA repeatedly stop breathing, or experience shallow breathing (hypopnea) during sleep. This can happen as often as three hundred times a night and can disrupt a person's quantity and quality of sleep. It is the partial collapse of the airway (the breathing tube between the nose, mouth, and lungs) that causes snoring, and it is the complete collapse that is the immediate cause of apnea. A study published in the *American Journal of Epidemiology* (2004) suggests that sleep-disordered breathing promotes glucose intolerance.

Correcting Sleep Apnea and Snoring

Sleep apnea and loud snoring may be another detrimental result of our Western lifestyle. The most important factors in correcting disordered breathing are losing weight, eliminating sugar, and other high-glycemic carbs from the diet, refraining from or stopping smoking, and avoiding alcohol. If you follow the dietary suggestions in Chapters 5 and 6, you can be on your way to correcting glucose metabolism and insulin resistance, which are implicated in this sleep disorder.

In the meantime, however, here are some ways to help reverse sleep apnea and snoring.

Lose weight. Excessive weight due to a sedentary lifestyle, too many rich foods, not sleeping well, and medically related conditions such as thyroid problems, are among the leading factors contributing to OSA. Spouses often make the observation that the larger their snoring spouse became, the louder the snoring bellowed, and the more often they heard snoring pauses followed by snorts and a resumption of breathing. Conversely, in a large percentage of patients, weight loss aided by exercise has reversed OSA.

Stop smoking. We are all aware that smoking has numerous undesirable effects on the body, but pertinent to OSA is the fact that cigarette smoking causes swelling of the mucous membranes in the nostrils, swelling of the tissue in the throat, and blockage of small vessels in the lungs, all of which can directly cause snoring and sleep apnea.

Avoid alcohol. Alcohol causes too great a relaxation of the airway during sleep, which contributes to loud snoring and sleep apnea.

Go to sleep and get up around the same time each day. Sleeping at irregular times can contribute to sleep-disordered breathing. It's important to go to bed and arise around the same time consistently. This is because there are two periods of sleep that are especially vulnerable to the development of unstable breathing: Stage 1 sleep, which should occur only when you're first falling asleep, but can occur many times during the night if sleep is poor; and REM sleep, when dreaming most frequently occurs.

Here's how irregular sleep times work: Say you go to bed at 10 PM and awaken at 6 AM each workday, but then wait until several hours later to go to sleep and wake up on weekend days. Both Stage 1 and REM sleep can behave oddly in this case. This problem with REM and Stage 1 is also true if on some days of the week you just don't get enough sleep, and then on other days of the week make up for it by sleeping much longer. The result in both cases can be the development of very significant respiratory instability during sleep. Correction of this problem requires stabilizing bedtime hours throughout the week.

Deal with blockages of the nose, throat, or lungs. Often nasal problems are caused by allergies to airborne particles, such as animal dander or dust, or to foods, which can cause swelling of the nasal passages; by dryness of the nose due to conditions such as a wood-burning stove; or by structural problems such as a deviated septum (the structure separating the left and right sides of the nose), in which airflow is blocked through one side. In that case, other structures in the nose (called turbinates) often grow larger on the unaffected side. The result can be almost complete blockage of nasal breathing. That, in turn, increases the effort the sleeper must make to breathe because of increased resistance to airflow, which can lead to OSA.

RESTLESS LEGS SYNDROME (RLS)

Restless legs syndrome (RLS) is a sleep disorder characterized by unpleasant sensations in the legs such as tingling, crawling, creeping, or pulling in the calf area. The feelings usually occur when you sit or lie down for long periods of time. To relieve the sensations, people with RLS have the urge to move their legs, making it difficult for them to relax and fall asleep.

Correcting RLS

Restless legs syndrome can develop as a result of certain biochemical conditions or nutrient deficiencies, including iron, folate, vitamin B_{12}, or magnesium.

Various substances can contribute to RLS. Avoid all xanthines (a purine-based compound found in certain plants), particularly coffee, cocoa, cola nut (used in cola drinks), chocolate, and black tea (herbal is fine). In one study, sixty-two patients with RLS showed signs of improvement on a xanthine-free diet. Also, avoid intake of alcohol and cigarette smoke. Be aware that certain drugs can cause RLS, including anticonvulsants such as methsuximide (Celontin Kapseals), phenytoin (Dilantin), antidepressants like amitriptyline HCl (Elavil) and paroxetine HCl (Paxil), beta-blockers, histamine-2 antagonists, lithium, and neuroleptics. Ask your doctor if any alternatives are available.

LACK OF EXPOSURE TO SUNLIGHT CAN CAUSE INSOMNIA

Most of us are undernourished when it comes to light. During the day, we receive diminished light from fluorescent bulbs rather than the vitamin-D-rich sunlight that our bodies crave. Then, during the night when we require darkness to trigger essential melatonin production, artificial light erodes our lunar consciousness and throws our body rhythms out of balance. In short, we have too much light when we don't need it at night, and too little of the right kind when we do need it during the day.

Researchers in Japan say lack of exposure to sunlight could explain why sleep disturbances are more common as people age. In a study of ten nursing home residents with insomnia, investigators found that increasing the residents' exposure to bright light increased their production of melatonin, a hormone that helps regulate sleep, and improved their sleeping patterns. Research has found that melatonin production declines with age.

The Japanese researchers exposed the patients to four hours of bright artificial light at midday for four weeks, roughly equal to the normal light exposure of the young control group. Investigators found that the extra light sent the elderly patients' melatonin production to a level similar to that of the young group and improved their sleep quality. Without their knowing exactly why, this may be one reason why many seniors move to sunny climates in their golden years.

A Simple Intervention for Lack of Light

To correct the problem of lack of exposure to sunlight, it is important to spend some time each day outside in the sun. You can walk, garden, bicycle, or do anything else you enjoy outside. During winter months when sunlight is limited, get full-spectrum lightbulbs for your home and office. And it's a good idea to take cod-liver oil during the winter, particularly for its vitamins A and D.

SHIFT WORK SLEEP DISORDER (SWSD)

Shift work sleep disorder is a sleep disorder that affects people who frequently rotate shifts or work at night. The natural sleep–wake cycle tells the body to sleep at night and be awake during the day, but this is disrupted for the shift worker. About 20 percent of the full-time workforce are shift workers, meaning they work more than half their hours outside the traditional work window of 6 AM to 6 PM. Working nights or rotating shifts puts people at risk for chronic sleep disruption; symptoms include excessive sleepiness when performing nighttime work and insomnia during daytime sleep opportunities.

Helpful Tips for SWSD

The following sleep tips for shift workers are adapted from those provided by the Mayo Clinic:

- Develop a pre-bedtime ritual. Read the paper, listen to soft music, or take a warm bath before going to bed. Allow yourself to unwind from your shift.
- Prepare your environment for sleeping. Sleep in a dark room. Use room-darkening shades or wear a sleep mask. Wear

earplugs or run a fan to block out daytime noises to make sleep easier.

- Maintain your sleep schedule. If at all possible, keep a consistent sleep schedule. Stick to the same sleep hours every day—even on your days off.
- Choose less frequent rotations. If possible, work a shift for three weeks rather than rotating to a different schedule every week.
- Change the sequence. A more normal sleep pattern results when your shift sequence is day–evening–night rather than day–night–evening.
- Take naps. A short nap—maybe thirty minutes—before your evening shift can help you feel refreshed and more alert at work. Rouse yourself well before your shift starts, though, in case you feel groggy when you first wake up.

MENOPAUSAL SLEEP PROBLEMS

Have you experienced more sleepless nights since entering menopause? It is very common for menopausal women to experience worsening sleep difficulties. "Postmenopausal women commonly report sleep problems," says Anne McTiernan of Fred Hutchinson Cancer Research Center in Seattle.

The National Sleep Foundation has reported that 20 percent of menopausal and postmenopausal women sleep less than six hours per night during the workweek, while only 12 percent of premenopausal women (with the exception of pregnant and menstruating women) sleep less than six hours. Among older women, lower levels of estrogen can cause problems with sleep. A lack of estrogen can also cause sleep-disturbing hot flashes and night sweats. Sleep deprivation can also cause women to suffer from memory disorders, concentration problems, anxiety, fatigue, muscle aches, and weight gain.

Correcting Menopausal Sleep Problems

- Avoid large meals, especially before bedtime. Also, some foods that are spicy or acidic may trigger hot flashes.
- Maintain a regular, normal weight.
- Avoid nicotine, caffeine, and alcohol, especially before bedtime.
- Dress in lightweight clothes to prevent overheating during the night. Avoid heavy, insulating blankets and comforters. A fan may be helpful to increase circulation.
- Avoid anything emotionally charging before bedtime, such as arguments or disturbing TV shows.
- Reduce stress and worry as much as possible. Try relaxation techniques, massage, and exercise. (See Chapter 3.)
- Unfortunately, hormone replacement therapy does not seem to help menopausal sleep problems. A study at the University of Michigan School of Nursing that was published in the *Journal of Women's Health* tested the connection between the hormone estrogen and women's sleep. Reseachers found that for women who were not having hot flashes, there was little difference in sleep between postmenopausal women who were taking estrogen supplements and those who were not. If you need hormones, seek out a holistic doctor who can prescribe natural hormones; they're much better for your overall health.

CHAPTER EIGHT ☽

The 21-Day Sleep Away the Pounds Menu Plan

The final step in the Sleep Away the Pounds Program is this exciting weight loss meal plan that will help you not only sleep better but also lose the weight you want. You'll kick off your new program with the 21-Day Sleep Away the Pounds Menu Plan. We think you'll be amazed at how you feel and look once you've been eating healthily for a couple of weeks—improved energy, loss of sugar cravings, better mood, weight loss, and definitely better sleep.

For the first twenty-one days you will eat healthy lean protein such as chicken, turkey, fish, beef, eggs, cheese, and nuts with lots of vegetables, leafy greens, low-sugar fruit, and good fats. You can choose good carbohydrates from a wide variety of brightly colored vegetables that are rich in antioxidants and other important vitamins and minerals that will support your immune system. Most of these foods you can eat as often as you like and as plentifully as you want. Lean meats, poultry, fish, eggs, cheese, and nuts will give your body the protein it needs. You can eat these foods in moderate portions.

Healthy fats such as fish oil, virgin coconut oil, and unrefined virgin olive oil will help satisfy your hunger. You need fat in your diet for satiety, that feeling of having had enough to eat. Virgin coconut oil also helps boost the body's metabolism. It burns quickly in the body, much like kindling in a fireplace, which promotes weight loss. It's the key ingredient in the recipes in our weight loss book *The Coconut Diet,* which has helped many people lose weight and improve their health. It also helps curb cravings, especially for sweets, and keeps hunger at bay. You may also enjoy unrefined virgin olive oil in salad dressings and drizzled over cold foods, along with small amounts of organic butter or ghee from grass-fed cows.

Grains processed into flour used in bread, bagels, muffins, rolls, buns, crackers, rice cakes, cereals, pasta, and pizza, along with white rice, should be avoided. You can have whole grains such as brown rice, quinoa, and amaranth. And there are a few breads that are truly whole grain, such as Ezekiel and manna bread. Alcohol (wine, beer, and liquor) and sweets are off the list, too—no cakes, cookies, pies, ice cream, doughnuts, or candy, along with higher-sugar fruit and high-starch vegetables such as potatoes and corn.

This is not a diet of deprivation, however, but one of enjoyment. With three meals per day and two snacks, you should not feel hungry or deprived. Best of all, you will learn a new style of eating that you can follow for the rest of your life.

Within days of starting this program, you should enjoy more energy, feel healthier, sleep better, and lose a couple of pounds. Some physical ailments may simply disappear. Three improvements that are often mentioned include more energy when you need it during the day, better mental clarity, and improved sleep. Many women note a significant reduction in PMS symptoms. And women who suffer from hot flashes often notice that they lessen. Joint problems get better for a lot of people. And scores of people who have suffered from low thyroid and adrenal dysfunction often experience exciting improvements.

You're not being asked to measure food or count carbs or calories with this diet—just choose from the lists of foods you can eat, and don't eat the foods on the "avoid" lists.

Low-carb eating, which is really low-sugar eating, will give your body a chance to deal with issues of insulin and leptin resistance brought on by eating too many of the wrong carbs, which are primarily the refined and processed ones. These foods not only pack on the pounds, but also can prevent you from sleeping well, because they are stimulating; they can also have an adverse effect on the endocrine system.

After several weeks on the Sleep Away the Pounds Diet, you should no longer experience swings in blood sugar. It will then be easier to control cravings for sweets and other high-glycemic foods. As a result, you will lose weight faster. And when your blood sugar is more stable and your endocrine glands such as your thyroid and adrenals are functioning better, you should sleep well all night.

When the three weeks are up, you should have lost your cravings for sweets, bread, starches, and alcohol. As a result, your body will be far less resistant to insulin and leptin and your blood sugar should be more stable. Best of all, you will be losing weight. And as an added bonus, your new lifestyle will help prevent serious diseases such as heart disease, cancer, obesity, and diabetes.

FOODS YOU CAN EAT

There's a wide array of delicious, healthy foods to choose from for your new Sleep Away the Pounds Menu Plan. Following are guidelines and lists of foods you can choose from to help you lose weight and gain sleep. You're on your way to a brand-new leaner you!

GUIDELINES FOR SERVINGS

Animal protein   4–6 ounces per meal

Eggs   No more than 2 per day

Legumes   3–4 1-cup servings per week

Grains   No more than 1 serving per day, but preferably not every day

Nuts, seeds, nut butters   24 small nuts such as almonds; 6 large nuts such as macadamias; 1 teaspoon nut butter per day

Low-sugar fruit   1–2 servings per day

Vegetables   Unlimited

Sweetener   Small amount of low-carb healthy sweetener

Water   At least 8 glasses pure water per day

Animal Proteins

Choose healthy, antibiotic-free (preferably organic and pasture-fed), lean cuts of meat and poultry in moderate portions. Between four and six ounces of animal protein is a healthy serving size. (A good visual is no larger than a deck of cards.)

Beef: Lean cuts of meat are best, such as:
　　Flank
　　New York
　　Sirloin
　　Tenderloin
　　Top round
　Bison (buffalo)
　Eggs
　Elk

Fish of all types
Lamb
Poultry:
    Chicken: Skinless breast and thighs are best
    Cornish game hens
    Turkey: Skinless is best
Turkey bacon (limit 2 slices)
Venison

Dairy

Choose antibiotic-free (preferably organic and pasture-fed) dairy products.

Cheese: Best choices are:
    Feta
    Goat cheese
    Mozzarella
    Ricotta
    Swiss

Beverages

Green tea or maté (omit if you have thyroid or adrenal gland dysfunction)
Herbal tea (hot and iced)
Mineral water with lemon or lime or unsweetened cranberry concentrate for flavor
Vegetable juices (fresh is best)

Grains and Cereal Grass

Brown rice
Oatmeal (not instant)

Quinoa
Whole grains such as barley, rye, and amaranth
Whole-grain breads such as Ezekiel and manna bread (other breads, though they may claim to be whole grain, and have some whole grain in them, are often mostly refined flour)
Wild rice (a cereal grass often thought of as a grain)

Eggs

Choose cage-free, preferably organic.

Fats and Oils

Butter (preferably organic and from pasture-fed cows)
Coconut oil (virgin is best)
Olive oil (unrefined extra virgin is best)

Fruit

Avocado
Apples
Berries:
  Blackberries
  Raspberries
  Blueberries
  Cranberries
Grapefruit
Lemon
Lime
Plums
Prunes
Strawberries

Nuts and Nut Butters; Seeds and Seed Butters

We recommend that you eat no more than the suggested single serving per day for maximum weight loss. If you combine nuts and seeds, keep the serving size in mind because nuts and seeds have carbohydrates, as well as protein and fat, and can cause weight gain.

Almonds (no more than 2 dozen)
Almond butter (1 tsp.)
Brazil nuts (no more than 6)
Cashews (no more than 6)
Cashew butter (1 tsp.)
Hazelnuts (no more than 12)
Hazelnut butter (1 tsp.)
Macadamia nuts (no more than 12)
Macadamia nut butter (1 tsp.)
Peanuts (actually not a nut—a legume) (no more than 24 small; avoid if you have low thyroid)
Peanut butter (1 tsp.; avoid if you have low thyroid)
Pecan halves (no more than 12)
Pine nuts (no more than 24)
Pistachios (no more than 24)
Pumpkin seeds (no more than 2 tbsp.)
Sesame seeds (no more than 2 tbsp.)
Sunflower seeds (no more than 2 tbsp.)
Tahini (sesame seed butter) (1 tsp.)
Walnut halves (no more than 12)

Note: You may have two or three dehydrated vegetable or seed crackers per day in place of nuts or seeds, depending on the ingredients; most of them have vegetable fiber added. Seed crackers are dehydrated and considered a raw food; they are made without any grains. Some health food stores carry them. You can also make them in a dehydrator. Almost all raw food recipe books have recipes for dehydrated crackers.

Sweeteners

Birch sugar (xylitol)
Lo Han Guo
Stevia

Vegetables and Legumes

Artichokes
Asparagus
Bamboo shoots
Beans:
    Aduki
    Black
    Butter
    Garbanzo
    Green and yellow wax
    Kidney
    Lentils
    Lima
    Split peas
Beets and beet greens
Bok choi
Broccoflower
Broccoli
Broccolini
Broccoli rabe
Brussels sprouts

Cabbage
    Chinese
    Green
    Red
    Savoy
Carrots
Cassava
Cauliflower
Celeriac
Celery
Chard
Chayote
Collards
Cucumber
Dandelion greens
Eggplant
Endive
Fennel
Jicama
Kale
Kohlrabi
Lettuce: All varieties, which include:
    Bibb/Boston
    Greenleaf
    Iceberg
    Redleaf
    Romaine
    Spring greens/mesclun
Mushrooms: All varieties, which include:
    Oyster
    Portobello
    Shiitake

Straw

Whole button

Mustard greens

Okra

Onions

Parsley

Pea pods

Peas

Peppers:

Green

Purple

Red

Yellow

Radicchio

Radishes

Rutabaga

Sauerkraut

Scallions

Sorrel

Spinach

Sprouts

Squash:

Butternut

Hubbard

Spaghetti

Summer/yellow

Zucchini

Swiss chard

Taro

Tomatillo

Tomatoes (considered a vegetable; actually a fruit, classified a berry): All varieties, which include:

    Cherry
    Plum
    Red (includes beefsteak)
    Roma
    Sun-dried
    Yellow pear
Turnips
Water chestnuts
Watercress

CHOOSING THE BEST

In the pages that follow, you'll discover which foods are the most nourishing for your body. It's the best food choices that will promote your best health and most restful sleep. It's well worth it to eat the best food, because when you're rested and well nourished, you'll have hardly any food cravings, less temptation to binge, and fewer urges to overeat. With your appetite under control, you'll lose weight faster and with far less struggle.

Animal Protein

Choose free-range, grass-fed beef and lamb whenever possible. You will not get appreciable amounts of CLA (conjugated linoleic acid) from meat unless you buy grass-fed dairy cow, beef, and lamb products. The body cannot produce CLA; we must get it from our food. CLA has been shown to promote weight loss.

    Whenever possible, shop for antibiotic-free and preferably organically raised lamb, beef, and poultry. The growth hormones injected into factory-farm-raised animals cause them to gain weight. After all, fattening animals quickly to get them to market means more dollars for the vendors. But what does it mean for us? These hormones are not healthful, and it's best to avoid them.

Natural-food markets such as Whole Foods, Wild Oats, local co-ops, and many independent health food stores as well as local farmers' markets offer grass-fed or naturally raised beef, lamb, buffalo, and poultry. Also, look for eggs from chickens that are raised cage-free, without hormones, and fed an organic diet. Finally, when you buy dairy products such as cheese, milk, and cream, get only organic products from grass-fed cows. These CLA-rich foods will facilitate weight loss.

Eggs are an excellent protein source and the best are cage-free, organically fed. They contain all eight essential amino acids and are a rich source of essential fatty acids. They also contain considerably more lecithin (a fat emulsifier) than cholesterol, and they are rich in sulfur and glutathione.

When it comes to fish, buy wild-caught. Farm-raised fish get treated almost as poorly as factory-farm-raised animals. They are often given antibiotics, raised penned in crowded pools, and not fed their customary marine diet. Hence, they do not have the essential fatty acids that wild-caught fish offer, which are so important for our health. This probably accounts for why their rather gray-colored flesh is dyed red before they're taken to market.

Quality lean protein is important for our health and weight management. It stimulates the production of glucagon, a hormone that functions opposite insulin. (Insulin will decrease secretion of glucagon.) Glucagon stabilizes blood sugar levels and provides brain fuel by signaling the body to release stored energy. When synchronized, insulin and glucagon create a stable hormonal system. But keep in mind that you can get too much animal protein, which is taxing for the kidneys and can contribute to overacidity in the system. That's why it's best to limit portion sizes to between four and six ounces.

When it comes to animal fat, fish is a good source of omega-3 fatty acids, especially wild-caught fatty cold-water fish such as salmon, mackerel, and trout. In general, though, keep animal fat to a minimum. Animals are higher on the food chain and tend to store toxins more often in fat cells rather than the muscle. Though organically raised animal products are far superior to those from factory-farm-raised animals, which are grown in penned, caged, or crowded, unhealthy conditions and given antibiotics, environmental toxins will still be stored in their fat.

Beverages

Green tea is especially helpful for weight loss. Not only is it rich in antioxidants—catechins and other polyphenols that protect us against inflammation, cancer, and other ailments—it is also a thermogenic. *Thermogenesis* means "production of heat," which revs up your metabolism. Most of the thermogenic action in green tea is due to epigallocatechin gallate (EGCG), which is a potent polyphenol. EGCG also appears to increase the effectiveness of weight loss supplements such as 5-HTP and tyrosine. For this reason, green tea is recommended as part of your daily meal plan. Strive for at least one cup of green tea per day. Avoid green tea, however, if you are caffeine-sensitive, have low adrenal or thyroid function, or are hypoglycemic. A cup of green tea has about a third of the caffeine found in a cup of coffee. When choosing green and herbal tea, look for the healthiest, which is organically grown. Also, unbleached tea bags are better choices than bleached.

Sparkling mineral water that is naturally carbonated, rather than commercially gassed, is best. Look for brands such as S. Pellegrino and Apollinaris.

Freshly made vegetable juice from organic produce is always a healthy choice. When choosing canned or bottled juices, choose low-sodium and organic, if available.

It is recommended that you drink at least eight 8-ounce glasses of water per day for any weight loss program; purified water is best.

A hydrated body is a healthy body. And for weight loss, plenty of water is very important. If you aren't drinking adequate amounts of water, your body will tend to hold on to it, and you could gain water weight.

Fats and Oils

The oils that are best for food preparation include virgin coconut oil, unrefined extra-virgin olive oil, ghee, and organic butter from grass-fed cows. You can use unrefined peanut, sesame, almond, and macadamia nut oils in small amounts for special dishes. Avoid all other oils.

Coconut oil. Be choosy when it comes to your coconut oil. Many commercial-grade coconut oils are made from copra, the dried kernel (meat) of the coconut. If standard copra is used as a starting material, the unrefined coconut oil extracted from it is not suitable for human consumption and must be refined. This is because most copra is dried under the sun in the open air in very unsanitary conditions where it is exposed to insects and molds. Though producers may start with organic coconuts and even label their coconut oil organic, the end product of some brands is refined, bleached, and deodorized to get rid of the molds and insects. High heat and chemical solvents are used in this process.

Olive oil is called virgin if it is extracted by means of pressure from millstones. Virgin olive oil is not treated with heat or chemicals. Batches of olives are pressed more than once to produce numerous batches of oil. The first pressing is the most flavorful and has the least acidity. The first cold pressing also has the greatest amount of fatty acids and polyphenols (antioxidants). Olive oils from the Mediterranean, and particularly Spain, are known to be the highest in antioxidants. The very best choice is extra-virgin, cold-pressed olive oil that is organically grown.

Butter. Unpasteurized butter from dairy cows that have been raised naturally and grass-fed is your best choice. This butter is rich in vitamins A and D and CLA. Use butter sparingly.

Ghee is a clarified butter without any solid milk particles or water. Ghee is used in India and throughout South Asia in daily cooking. Quality ghee adds a great aroma, flavor, and taste to food. According to ancient ayurvedic medicine, a moderate amount of ghee is the best cooking oil. Purchase only organic ghee made from dairy cows; completely avoid ghee made from vegetable oil. (Ghee made from diary cows can be found at many health food stores, natural markets, and Indian markets.)

Fruit, Vegetables, and Legumes

Fruit. One of the best fruits you can choose is avocado. It is an excellent source of essential fatty acids, glutathione (a powerful antioxidant), and protein. It contains more potassium than bananas (they're off the list because of their high sugar content), making them an excellent choice for those with heart disorders. Also, berries are an excellent choice because they are low in sugar and rich in antioxidants. Choose organically grown, low-sugar fruit. See the list of low-sugar fruits on page 169.

Vegetables. Most vegetables are on the list of foods you can enjoy. We encourage you to eat lots of them, as they're packed with satisfying, health-enhancing nutrients. Eat plenty of salads, sprouts, vegetable sticks, and steamed vegetables. High-starch vegetables such as potatoes and corn are off the list. If you are dining out or it's a special occasion and you just can't resist a potato, the best choice is red-skinned potatoes (fewer carbs). If you do succumb to a baked potato, which is very high in carbs, eat it with fat such as sour cream or butter. This will help to slow down the rate at which sugar enters your bloodstream. Avoid mashed potatoes, which turn to sugar very rapidly in the bloodstream, or if you just can't resist, take only a few bites and leave the rest. This is only for special occasions.

Legumes. The outer casing of legumes (the fiber) slows down the rate at which sugar enters your bloodstream. You can choose beans, lentils, or split peas. While you're working on losing weight, it's best to limit legumes to three to four 1-cup servings a week for the first three weeks due to their carb content.

Organic produce. Choose organic produce as often as possible to avoid toxic pesticides. In 1995, the USDA tested nearly seven thousand fruit and vegetable samples and detected residues of sixty-five different pesticides, with two out of three samples containing pesticide residue.

Plants absorb nutrients from the soil—and they also take up pesticides. Healthy soil is rich in minerals and alive with micro-organisms. Pesticides kill these much-needed minute organisms. Additionally, chemical fertilizers do not replenish the soil in any manner close to traditional composting and other natural practices that nourish soil.

The quality of protein in grains and vegetables is related to the amount of nitrogen in the soil. When a lot of nitrogen is present, plants increase protein production and decrease carbohydrate synthesis. When their metabolic protein requirements are satisfied, what remains is stored in the form of protein that contains fewer essential amino acids. This means that the result of high levels of nitrogen, as found in conventional chemical fertilizers, is an increase in the amount of protein but a reduction in its quality. Organically managed, composted soils release nitrogen in smaller amounts over a longer time than conventional fertilizers. As a result, the quality of protein from organic crops is better in terms of human nutrition.

While organic foods are always the best option in terms of

avoiding pesticides, studies show they are also higher in nutrient content. In a 2001 study published in the *Journal of Complementary and Alternative Medicine,* on average, organic produce contained 27 percent more vitamin C, 21 percent more iron, and 29 percent more magnesium than conventional produce, and all twenty-one minerals compared in the study were higher in the organic produce.

The more nutrient-rich foods you eat, the more your body will be satisfied and cravings will diminish. In this respect, organic produce is helpful for weight loss. But the most important reason to choose organically grown food is for your health.

Salt

Sea salt or Celtic salt, also known as gray salt, is the best choice. Whole sea salt has a mineral profile similar to that of our blood. Regular table salt is a highly refined product; when it's processed, minerals are removed, and what remains is sodium chloride. Anticaking chemicals, potassium oxide, iodine, and dextrose (sugar) are added to make table salt. If you need to avoid excess trace minerals for medical reasons, then choose kosher salt, which is simply pure sodium chloride.

Spice Up Your Meals!

Black pepper, cayenne, ginger, and turmeric all have been shown to induce thermogenesis, which means they help you metabolize fat. You can add them often to your favorite recipes. Not only will you assist your body in burning fat, but you'll also help prevent some diseases such as cancer.

Sweeteners

There are three low-carb healthy sweeteners recommended: stevia, birch sugar (xylitol), and Lo Han Guo.

Birch sugar (xylitol) is a sugar alcohol. The healthiest xylitol is derived from birch bark. It has fewer calories than sugar with about the same sweetness. It has not been shown to promote tooth decay, and it is metabolized slowly, which helps prevent the sugar highs and lows often experienced with other sweeteners. Keep in mind that not all xylitol may be derived from birch bark and may not be as healthy.

Substances such as sorbitol, manitol, malitol, and xylitol are sugar alcohols that are derived from dextrose or glucose, or—in the case of xylitol—from birch trees or a by-product of the paper industry. The labels of gums and candies containing these ingredients may say "sugar-free," but this is somewhat misleading—when broken down, sugar alcohols act similarly to other forms of sugar. None is free of calories, and only xylitol does not promote cavities. These products tend to ferment in the digestive tract, causing cramping and diarrhea. As already stated, the best sugar alcohol is xylitol, derived from birch trees. Our favorite is the Ultimate Sweetener, which is made from Finnish birch bark.

Lo Han Guo comes from the Chinese plant Lo Han Guo (*Siraitia grosvenorii*), a perennial vine in the cucumber or melon family that grows in China. Lo Han Guo fruits contain a triterpene glycoside sweetener known as mogroside. When processed into a fine powder, this natural sweetener is soluble in water. It is about three hundred times sweeter than sugar, so very little is needed to sweeten foods and beverages. It is also very low in calories.

Stevia is extracted from the herbal leaf of a plant that grows in South America. Like Lo Han Guo, it is two to three hundred times sweeter than sugar, so you need only a small amount in comparison. It has virtually no calories. There is no evidence that it is harmful to the body in any way. The FDA does not allow it to be marketed as a sweetener, so it's labeled as a nutritional supplement. Stevia comes in powdered or liquid form and can be found at most health food stores.

GLYCEMIC INDEX AND GLYCEMIC LOAD

The best diet for weight loss and better sleep is a low-sugar diet. Therefore, it is advantageous to understand the glycemic index (GI) and the meaning of glycemic load (GL) and to especially avoid foods with a high GI or GL.

The glycemic index is a numerical system of measuring the rise in circulating blood sugar that is triggered by a carbohydrate. Therefore, the higher the GI number, the greater the blood sugar response. A low-GI food will cause a small rise in blood sugar, while a high-GI food will trigger a dramatic spike. The GI of foods is based on glucose that is set to equal 100. A GI of 70 or more is considered high, a GI of 56 to 69 is medium, and a GI of 55 or less is low. A list of foods and their glycemic values can be found in a variety of books (try *The New Glucose Revolution Complete Guide to Glycemic Index Values* by Jennie Brand-Miller) and on Web sites such as www.mendosa.com/gilists.htm.

The glycemic load is a relatively new way to assess the impact of carbohydrate consumption that takes the glycemic index into account, but gives a more complete picture than does the GI alone. A GI value tells you only how rapidly a particular carbohydrate turns into sugar. It doesn't tell you how much of that carbohydrate is in a serving of a particular food. You need to know both values to understand a food's effect on blood sugar. That's where glycemic load comes in. The GL is the GI divided by 100 multiplied by its available carbohydrate content (for example, carbohydrates minus fiber) in grams. The carbohydrate in watermelon, for example, has a high GI. But there isn't a lot of it, so watermelon's GL is relatively low. A GL of 20 or more is high, a GL of 11 to 19 is medium, and a GL of 10 or less is low.

Foods that have a low GL almost always have a low GI value. But foods with an intermediate or high GL can range from very low to very high GI. Some lists such as the Web site www.mendosa.com/gilists.htm include both GI and GL.

Agave syrup. The agave plant is cultivated in hilly, semi-arid soils of Mexico. Its fleshy leaves contain a sweet, sticky juice (or nectar), which is about 90 percent fructose. Only recently has it come into use as a sweetener. It has a low glycemic index and is a delicious and safe alternative to table sugar. Unlike the crystalline form of fructose, which is refined primarily from corn, agave syrup is fructose in its natural form and does not contain processing chemicals. Even better, because fructose is sweeter than table sugar, less is needed in your recipes. It can be very useful for people who are diabetic, have insulin or leptin resistance, or are simply watching their carbohydrate intake.

Though fructose has a low glycemic value, according to some experts, if it is consumed after eating a large meal that overly raises the blood sugar or with high-glycemic foods, it no longer has a low glycemic value. Strangely enough, it will take on the value of the higher-glycemic food. So exercise restraint.

FOODS TO AVOID

Animal Proteins

Fatty cuts of beef (avoid for best weight loss results and better health—more toxins are stored in fat than muscle); these include:
   Brisket
   Liver
   Liverwurst
   Ribs
   Rib-eye steak
Pork in general, but especially avoid:
   Bacon
   Honey-baked ham

Poultry:
    Duck
    Goose
    Processed poultry products

Beverages

Alcohol: Beer, liquor, wine
Anything with artificial flavors or sweeteners
Chocolate drinks/cocoa
Coffee/coffee drinks
Fruit juice
Regular and diet sodas
Sports drinks

Dairy and Milk Substitutes

Cheeses that are processed
Dairy creamer substitutes
Ice cream
Soy milk (a goitrogen; not recommended for thyroid health)
Yogurt that is sweetened

Fats

Commercial salad dressings made with any of the oils listed
    below
Margarine
Polyunsaturated oils:
    Corn
    Safflower
    Soybean
    Sunflower

Fruit

Bananas
Dates
Figs
Papaya
Pineapple
Raisins

Grain Products

Bagels
Biscuits
Bread
Bread sticks
Breakfast pastries
Buns
Cereals
Cereal bars
Crackers
Doughnuts
English muffins
Muffins
Pancakes
Pasta
Pizza dough
Rolls
Stuffing
Tortillas
Waffles

Snack Foods

Cheese snacks
Chips:
    Corn
    Potato
    Tortilla
Popcorn
Pretzels
Soy crisps and snacks
Vegetable chips and snacks

Sweets

Barbecue sauce with sweetener
Desserts:
    Brownies
    Cakes
    Candy
    Cookies
    Frozen yogurt
    Gelatin
    Ice cream
    Mousse
    Pies
    Pudding
    Sorbet
    Whipped topping
Energy bars
Jams
Jellies
Ketchup
Syrup

Sugar
   Brown
   Maple
   Powdered
   White
Sweeteners
   All artificial sweeteners, including aspartame (NutraSweet)
      and sucralose (Splenda)
   Brown rice syrup
   Honey
   Molasses

Vegetables

Corn
Potatoes: All varieties, which include:
   Idaho
   New white
   Red-skinned

JUICING FOR WEIGHT LOSS

Vegetable juice (not fruit juice) is excellent for weight loss. It is packed with appetite-suppressing soluble fiber and replete with nutrients, which help you start your day satisfied so you won't be craving something decadent midmorning. A great asset in peeling off the pounds! Fat cells respond to starvation by holding on to fat. This is one of the body's systems designed to keep us alive in times of famine. Vegetable juice offers an abundance of nutrients that feed our bodies superior nutrition without a lot of calories.

When you skip breakfast or other meals, a signal is sent to your body that it's starving. This causes it to store or hold on to fat for further use. Fresh vegetable juice in the morning provides your body with a host of nutrients and enzymes that send a signal that it's well fed, and they supercharge your brain so you can function better all morning. Juice is known as a "live food," meaning that it hasn't had its vitamins and enzymes destroyed by heat or processing—it's alive with nutrients! When your cells are well fed with nutrients, you will have the energy to meet the day's demands.

A glass of fresh vegetable juice each day can help you power-pack your day with nutrients your body can use, as opposed to empty calories your body can't use and will tend to store in fat cells, such as a bowl of sugary flakes. You can take fresh juice to work in a thermos, or drink it before you leave home. It's fabulous in providing energizing nutrients that tell your body: *You aren't hungry anymore!*

You'll need a good juicer if you want to make sure juicing fits into your lifestyle. If you don't have a good juicer, choose one that is easy to clean, is stainless steel, and has a good motor (half a horsepower).

THE FAST-TRACK 1-DAY JUICE CLEANSE

You may want to try the 1-Day Vegetable Juice Cleanse for one, two, or all three weeks. This is an optional all-liquid day that helps facilitate faster weight loss. You might prefer to choose a weekend or other day when you don't have to work outside your home, which makes it easier to incorporate, but you can make this day happen at work by taking the juices to work in a thermos. During the day, you will only drink vegetable juices, vegetable broth, water, sparkling mineral water, and herbal or green teas. That's all. This day is a great boost to weight loss and will especially help you get rid of excess stored water and toxins. It also helps to rejuvenate the body, jump-start your weight loss program, and push you over a weight loss plateau.

The 1-Day Juice Fast Menu

Breakfast
Herbal or green tea with lemon juice *or*
Hot water with lemon and a dash of cayenne pepper *and*
Vegetable juice of choice

Morning
9:30 AM   8 ounces water
10:30 AM   Herbal tea, green tea, *or* vegetable juice
11:30 AM   8 ounces water *or* sparkling mineral water*

Lunch
Vegetable juice

Afternoon
1:30 PM   8 ounces still water *or* sparkling mineral water
2:30 PM   8 ounces still water *or* sparkling mineral water
3:00 PM   Herbal tea, green tea, warm vegetable broth, *or* vegetable juice
4:00 PM   8 ounces still water *or* sparkling mineral water
5:00 PM   8 ounces still water *or* sparkling mineral water

Dinner
8–10 ounces vegetable juice of choice *or*
Vegetable juice or cold soup made with fresh veggie juice and blended with an avocado (you may also add a cup of warm vegetable broth)

Sparkling mineral water may be substituted for water at any time. You may add a squeeze of lemon or lime for added flavor, or a dash of unsweetened cranberry juice.

THE 21-DAY SLEEP AWAY THE POUNDS MENU PLAN

Your 21-Day Sleep Away the Pounds Menu Plan is designed to facilitate healthy weight loss and restful sleep. It will help you meet your nutritional needs and not feel deprived. Best of all, you'll learn a new way of eating that will help you keep weight off for good!

Basic Guidelines

Drink at least eight glasses of water each day. The current recommendation from many holistic doctors is that you drink one quart of water for each fifty pounds of body weight. So if you weigh more than a hundred pounds, you should be drinking more than eight glasses of water a day. We recommend purified water. Drinking adequate water will facilitate weight loss. Sometimes we think we're hungry when we're actually thirsty, so before you eat anything, drink a glass of water. Then see if you're still hungry.

Design your weight loss program to meet your particular needs. The 21-Day Menu Plan serves as a guideline. You may pick and choose what fits your lifestyle. The important thing is that you avoid the carbohydrates and other foods that are listed on the "avoid" list.

When eating out, say "No bread please." It helps when dining in restaurants to tell your server not to bring bread to the table. Order hamburgers without the bun and sandwiches without the bread. This will help eliminate a lot of fattening carbs.

DAY ONE ──────────────────────

BREAKFAST

Green or herbal tea with a slice of lemon
6–8 ounces vegetable juice, preferably fresh
Scrambled eggs
1 slice turkey bacon
2 slices fresh tomato sprinkled with fresh or dried herbs of choice
   and a dash of sea salt

MIDMORNING BREAK

Green or herbal tea with lemon
6 raw or toasted almonds

LUNCH

Baked fish with steamed vegetables and ¼ cup wild rice

MIDAFTERNOON SNACK

Sparkling mineral water with a slice of lemon
1 stalk celery stuffed with soft goat cheese, cut into 6 pieces

DINNER

Chicken Caesar salad and a cup of soup

DAY TWO ──────────────────────

BREAKFAST

Green or herbal tea with lemon
6–8 ounces vegetable juice, preferably fresh
Oatmeal (not instant) with berries and milk of choice

MIDMORNING BREAK

Green or herbal tea
A piece of fruit

LUNCH

Vegetable soup and green salad

MIDAFTERNOON SNACK

Herbal tea (iced or hot) with a slice of lemon
6 raw or toasted almonds

DINNER

Vegetable stir-fry with organic tofu
Garden salad

DAY THREE

BREAKFAST

Green or herbal tea with lemon
Cheese omelet with sautéed vegetables

MIDMORNING BREAK

6–8 ounces vegetable juice, preferably fresh
1 celery stalk stuffed with 1 teaspoon almond butter, cut into
6 pieces

LUNCH

Cup of gazpacho
Hamburger patty with lettuce, tomato, onion, and pickle, no bun;
mustard or mayo, as desired

MIDAFTERNOON SNACK

Sparkling mineral water with a slice of lime or lemon
2 slices deli turkey or roast beef

DINNER

Beans and brown rice with mixed green salad of cucumber,
tomato, green onions, and grated carrot with vinaigrette

DAY FOUR

BREAKFAST

Green or herbal tea with lemon
Smoked salmon and sliced tomatoes with fresh basil and a
sprinkle of sea salt

MIDMORNING BREAK

1 hard-boiled egg
6–8 ounces vegetable juice, preferably fresh

LUNCH

Bean or lentil soup and salad

MIDAFTERNOON SNACK

3–4 sardines, packed in mustard sauce

DINNER

Turkey breast and steamed vegetables
Sliced tomatoes with fresh or dried herbs of choice and a sprinkle
of sea salt

DAY FIVE

BREAKFAST

Green or herbal tea with lemon
6–8 ounces vegetable juice, preferably fresh
Crustless quiche or egg bake

MIDMORNING BREAK

Herbal tea (iced or hot)
6 macadamia nuts

LUNCH

Chili with beans, mildly spicy

Mixed green salad

MIDAFTERNOON SNACK

Sparkling mineral water with a slice of lemon

2–3 slices deli turkey

DINNER

Main-course salad with grilled salmon

Cup of soup

DAY SIX

BREAKFAST

Green or herbal tea with lemon

6–8 ounces vegetable juice, preferably fresh

Amaranth, millet, or oatmeal with berries and milk of choice

MIDMORNING BREAK

1 stalk celery stuffed with soft goat cheese, cut into 6 pieces

LUNCH

Spinach salad or Cobb salad

Cup of soup

MIDAFTERNOON SNACK

3–4 sardines packed in mustard sauce

DINNER

Baked fish

Steamed green beans

Wild rice (¼ cup)

Green salad with vinaigrette and sesame or sunflower seeds sprinkled on top

DAY SEVEN

BREAKFAST

Green or herbal tea with lemon
2 soft-boiled eggs
2 slices turkey bacon

MIDMORNING BREAK

Vegetable sticks with herbed mayonnaise or salad dressing

LUNCH

Hummus with veggie sticks
Cucumber salad

MIDAFTERNOON SNACK

6–8 ounces vegetable juice, preferably fresh

DINNER

Quinoa or brown rice and steamed vegetables
Crispy green salad with olive-oil-and-vinegar dressing

Repeat this style of eating for two more weeks. Hopefully, at the end of the three weeks you will be sleeping well, losing weight, and enjoying a new style of eating that can be yours for life.

DINNERS THAT HELP YOU SLEEP

Meals that are rich in complex carbohydrates and tryptophan, but low to medium in protein, will help you relax in the evening and set you up for a good night's sleep. Try the following dinners to help you sleep:

- Turkey with vegetables, especially dark green veggies
- Scrambled eggs with veggies and cheese
- Tofu stir-fry
- Beans and brown rice with a leafy green salad
- Hummus with vegetable sticks and sliced cucumber salad
- Chicken Caesar salad
- Chili with beans, mildly spicy, and a leafy green salad
- Sesame or sunflower seeds sprinkled on a salad with turkey or chicken chunks
- Navy bean soup with a leafy green salad
- Fish and steamed vegetables

Eat lighter meals for dinner. Eating lighter in the evening is more likely to give you a restful night's sleep. High-fat meals and large servings prolong the work of your digestive system and may keep you awake. For most people, going to bed with a full stomach does not promote a restful night's sleep. While you may fall asleep faster, all the intestinal work required to digest a big meal is likely to cause frequent awakenings and a poorer quality of sleep. You may also find that heavily seasoned foods (hot peppers, spices) interfere with sleep as do dessert, coffee, and alcohol. It's also best to eat your evening meal before 7 PM.

CONCLUSION

Summing It Up, Sending You Off!

Now that you've read *Sleep Away the Pounds*, you're all set to embark on the most comprehensive weight loss program available. The four easy steps of the Sleep Away the Pounds Program begin with a good night's sleep. Step One is one of the most important and—until now—the most overlooked step in the weight loss process. Step Two helps you quiet your mind and calm your soul so you can truly rest and balance your appetite-influencing hormones while you sleep. To that end, you've learned how to relax and reduce stress and how to nourish your body, soul, and spirit. Step Three gets you up on your feet and moving your body as you improve your muscle tone and metabolism for more efficient weight loss and naturally better sleep. Step Four guides you in food choices that help you choose the best calories for weight loss and the finest food for a night of refreshing sleep.

It's all here in the revolutionary Sleep Away the Pounds Weight Loss Program. It's the one that offers you the very best chance at losing weight—whether you've struggled for years to shed pounds or you just decided you'd like to lose some weight. You now know from the research that it all starts with balancing your hormones, so that the hormones that curb your appetite can help you control the hormones that make you crave rich, fattening foods. By getting a good night's sleep, you'll have the very best chance of controlling your hunger. This will enable you to make wise food choices and not feel overwhelmed by cravings. As you put into practice the tips for getting the best sleep possible, you'll be on your way to looking younger (what they say about beauty sleep is true!), healthier, and leaner than ever.

We want you to sleep well and eat well for the rest of your life. As you do, gone will be the days of frustration over unwanted pounds. We wish you restful nights and centered days, and we send you off to sleep away all the unwanted pounds.

THE COMPLETE PRESCRIPTION FOR THE SLEEP AWAY THE POUNDS PROGRAM

Step One: Sleep

- Sleep an additional thirty minutes whenever possible.
- Get seven to nine hours of sleep, unless you need more or less.
- Determine your sleep needs (see page 8).
- Get the most restorative, refreshing sleep possible.

Step Two: Reduce Stress, Restore Your Soul

- Pick at least one stress-reduction exercise that will help you keep stress under control and quiet your mind at night.
- Each day, make time to restore your soul through meditation, prayer, or any other means you wish, to let go of worries, anxieties, and stressful thoughts and renew your mind and emotions.

- Schedule time each week to have fun. Do something that is truly enjoyable for you and forget about everything stressful during this time.
- Get away for a day or a weekend several times a year and do something relaxing.
- Take a vacation at least once a year and get away from everything stressful including telephones, e-mails, and anything else connected to work.
- Visit a health spa or get a massage.
- Practice appreciation and live from a thankful heart. It's a powerful way to combat stress.

Step Three: Exercise
- Pick one form of aerobic exercise that you will do at least three times a week.
- Pick one method of strength training that you will incorporate into your regimen each week.
- Choose a stretching/breathing routine that you will include every week in your exercise program.

Step Four: Eat Well
- Follow the low-sugar diet.
- Include plenty of omega-3-rich foods, such as fish, leafy green vegetables, seeds, and nuts.
- Eat lots of brightly colored vegetables and low-sugar fruit.
- Avoid foods such as coffee, alcohol, and refined carbs that keep you awake and pack on the pounds.
- Avoid all artificial foods such as substitute sweeteners, fake fats, and artificial flavors and additives.
- Include supplements that help you sleep and promote weight loss.

ACKNOWLEDGMENTS

To those who assisted us in researching and writing, we are forever grateful. Michele Libin, you are a dear friend and a valued writer with a wonderful future ahead in writing; thank you for your contribution to Chapter Four. Heather King, you are very professional and have a great future ahead as you graduate from Bastyr University, for you're a very good writer and well-trained nutritionist; thank you for your contribution to Chapter Three. To Nina Watkins, MS, LAc, acupuncturist at Balanced Health Acupuncture, thank you for writing the informative section on acupuncture for Chapter Seven. To our dear friend Dr. Bob Whitehouse, thank you so much for sharing sleep tips you designed for your clientele; you've always been so generous. And to Dr. Matthew Nash, DC, chiropractor at Nash Chiropractic, thank you for contributing the section on chiropractics for Chapter Seven.

To our editors Diana Baroni and Leila Porteous who made this project happen, thank you for your creativity and determination to make this book the very best it could be.

We also thank our lovely literary agent Pamela Harty, who continues to help us find a home for our work.

Lastly, we wish to express our deep and lasting appreciation to all the people, the Holy Trinity, and the angels who have assisted us with this book. To our dear heavenly Father, Savior, Jesus Christ, and Holy Spirit, thank you for guiding us throughout this project to discover more information than we ever dreamed we'd find to help people sleep well. Thank you for showing us Your ways, wisdom, and truth. And thank you, too, for the tough times while working on this project; sleepless nights like we'd never known before that gave us great empathy for those who can't sleep well. Thank you for our health and the awesome responsibility of guiding those who have lost their health, peace of mind, restful sleep, or their way concerning the care of their bodies. For the healing You've given us and Your unconditional love, we are so very appreciative.

—Cherie and John Calbom

RESOURCES

WEB SITES FOR CHERIE AND JOHN CALBOM

www.sleepawaythepounds.com: Information about the Sleep Away the Pounds Program and products, as well as "Precious Sleep" information and products. You can call 1-866-8GETWEL (1-866-843-8935).

www.gococonuts.com: Information about the Coconut Diet and coconut oil.

www.juicinginfo.net: Information about juicing and juicers.

www.wrinklecleanse.com: Information about the Wrinkle Cleanse.

www.ultimatesmoothie.com: Information about *The Ultimate Smoothie Book* and healthy smoothies.

www.cancercleanse.net: Information about *The Complete Cancer Cleanse* book.

www.cheriecalbom.com: Information about the authors and their books and other Web sites.

OTHER BOOKS BY CHERIE AND JOHN CALBOM

These books can be ordered at any of the Web sites noted above or by calling 1-866-8GETWEL (1-866-843-8935).

The Wrinkle Cleanse (Avery) by Cherie Calbom.

The Coconut Diet (Warner) by Cherie Calbom and John Calbom.

The Complete Cancer Cleanse (Warner) by Cherie Calbom, John Calbom, and Michael Mahaffey.

The Ultimate Smoothie Book (Warner) by Cherie Calbom.

"Precious Sleep" information and products. You can call 1-866-8GETWEL (1-866-843-8935).

JUICERS, SMOOTHIE MAKERS, AND WATER PURIFIERS

Call 1-866-8GETWEL (1-866-843-8935) for recommendations by Cherie Calbom, or see www.sleepawaythepounds.com.

LYMPHASIZER

Call 1-866-8GETWEL (1-866-843-8935) or see www.sleepawaythepounds.com.

FOOD PRODUCTS

Coconut Oil
Call 1-866-8GETWEL (1-866-843-8935) or see www.sleepawaythepounds .com to order virgin coconut oil.

Sugar
Pure birch sugar: The Ultimate Sweetener is available at some health food stores, or call 1-800-843-6325.

CLEANSE PRODUCTS

Colon Cleanse
Advanced Naturals: Fiber Max, and Colon Cleanse I and II, are available at health food stores.
Arise & Shine Products: Psyllium, bentonite, herbal nutrition, and Chomper. Call 1-866-8GETWEL (1-866-843-8935) or see www.sleepawaythepounds.com.
Garden of Life: Super Seed (fiber only). Contact www.gardenoflifeusa.com or 1-800-622-8986.

Liver/Gallbladder Products

Livercleanse products (1-866-843-8935).
Metagenics: Lipo-Gen lipotropic formula. Call 1-866-8GETWEL (1-866-843-8935).

Kidney Cleanse Herbs
Arise & Shine: Kidney Life. Call 1-866-8GETWEL (1-866-843-8935).

Candida Cleanse Products
Garden of Life: Fungal Defense. Contact www.gardenoflifeusa.com or 1-800-622-8986.
Advanced Naturals: Yeast Max. Available at health food stores.
Flora Grow. Call 1-866-8GETWEL (1-866-843-8935).

Parasite Cleanse Products
Arise & Shine: Worm Squirm I and II. Call 1-866-8GETWEL (1-866-843-8935).

Probiotics
Garden of Life: Primal Defense. Contact www.gardenoflifeusa.com or 1-800-622-8986.

Juice Concentrates
Dynamic Health makes cranberry juice concentrates. Available at health food stores.

SUPPLEMENTS AND RELATED PRODUCTS

Sinupret: Call 1-800-264-2325.
GABA: Pain and Stress Center, San Antonio, Texas. Call 1-800-669-2256.

ADRENAL SUPPORT

Adrengen and Adreset (metagenics) see www.sleepawaythepounds.com or call 1-866-843-8935.
Standard Process: Desiccated Adrenal. Call 1-800-558-8740.
Biotics Research: Liquid Iodine. Available at some health food stores.

THYROID SUPPORT

Thyrosol (Metagenics): see www.sleepawaythepounds.com or call 1-866-8GETWEL (1-866-843-8935).

MINERALS

Eniva Essentials: Bio Available Liquid Minerals. Call 1-866-8GETWEL (1-866-843-8935).

SLEEP AIDS

See www.sleepawaythepounds.com or call 1-866-843-8935 for the best sleep aid recommendations.

HEALTH CENTERS

The following centers offer a raw foods/juice detoxification program. Most of them offer nutritional classes; some offer other health classes that address the emotional, mental, and spiritual aspects of health and renewal. Most also offer massage and colonics. It is best to contact the various centers to find out which one best fits your needs.

Cedar Springs Renewal Center

Michael Mahaffey and Nan Monk, Directors
31459 Barben Road
Sedro Woolley, WA 98284
(360) 826-3599
Fax (360) 422-1524
www.cedarsprings.org

HealthQuarters Ministries

David Frahm, ND, Director
3620 West Colorado Avenue
Colorado Springs, CO 80904
(719) 593-8694
Fax (719) 531-7884
healthqu@healthquarters.org
www.healthquarters.org

Hippocrates Institute

Brian and Anna Maria Clement, Directors
1443 Palmdale Court

West Palm Beach, FL 33411
(800) 842-2125
Fax (561) 471-9464
hippocrates@worldnet.att.net
www.hippocratesinstitute.org

Optimum Health Institute of Austin

Route 1, Box 339 J
Cedar Creek, TX 78612
(512) 303-4817
Fax (512) 303-1239
austin@optimumhealth.org
www.optimumhealth.org

Optimum Health Institute of San Diego

6970 Central Avenue
Lemon Grove, CA 91945
(800) 993-4325
Fax (619) 589-4098
optimum@optimumhealth.org
www.optimumhealth.org

Sanoviv Medical Institute

Dr. Myron Wentz, Director
Playa de Rosarito, Room 39
Baja California, Mexico
(800) 726-6848
Fax (801) 954-7477
www.sanoviv.com

We Care

Susana and Susan Lombardi, Directors
18000 Long Canyon Road
Desert Hot Springs, CA 92241
(800) 888-2523
Fax (760) 251-5399

info@wecarespa.com
www.wecarespa.com

INSOMNIA

National Women's Health Information Center. Call 1-800-994-9662.

National Center on Sleep Disorders Research (NCSDR) (NHLBI). Contact 301-435-0199 or www.nhlbi.nih.gov/sleep.

National Heart, Lung, and Blood Institute. Contact 301-592-8573 or www.nhlbi.nih.gov.

American Academy of Sleep Medicine. Contact 708-492-0930 or www.aasmnet.org.

National Sleep Foundation. Contact 202-347-3471 or www.sleepfoundation.org.

REFERENCES

CHAPTER ONE

Beers T. Flexible schedules and shift work: replacing the "9-to-5" workday? *Mon Labor Rev* 2000; 123:33–40.

Burgess H, Penev P, Schneider R, Van Cauter E. Estimating cardiac autonomic activity during sleep: impedance cardiography, spectral analysis, and Poincaré plots. *Clin Neurophys* 2004; 115:19–28.

Chronic insomnia shown to be a medical condition, not just loss of sleep. *J Clin Endocrinol Metab* 2001; 86:3787–3794. www.endosociety.org/news/press/2001.

Cobb K. Missed ZZZs. More Disease Science News Online, Sept. 2, 2002.

Desaulniers M. Stimulating the body's production of human growth hormone. www.bodybuildingforyou.com/articles-submit/mary-desaulniers.

Diagnostic and Statistical Manual of Mental Disorders, 4th ed. (Washington, DC: American Psychiatric Association, 2000).

Garcia J, Garcia-Touza M, Hijazi R, Taffet G, Epner D, Mann D, Smith R, Cunningham G, Marcelli M. Active ghrelin levels and active to total ghrelin ratio in cancer-induced cachexia. *J Clin Endocrinol Metab* 2005; 90:2920–2926. PMID 15713718.

Graci S. *The Food Connection* (Toronto: Macmillan, 2001), 43–44.

Hellmich N. Healthy weight might rest with diet, exercise, and sleep-linked hormones. *USA Today*, Dec. 7, 2004, 1–2D. www.usatoday.com/news/health/2004-12-06-sleep-weight-gain.

Insulin resistance and pre-diabetes. www.diabetes.niddk.nih.gov/dm/pubs/insulin resistance.

Kojima M, Hosoda H, Date Y, Nakazato M, Matsuo H, Kangawa K. Ghrelin is a growth-hormone-releasing acylated peptide from stomach. *Nature* 1999; 402:656–660. PMID 10604470.

Lambert C. Deep into sleep. www.harvardmagazine.com/on-line/070587.

Meerlo P et al. Sleep restriction alters the hypothalamic-pituitary-adrenal response to stress. *J Neuroendocrinol* 2002; 14:397–402.

Mercola J, Droege R. Is insomnia wreaking havoc on your health? www.mercola.com, Feb. 7, 2004.

NAASO, The Obesity Society. 2005 Annual meeting Tuesday highlights: low-tech weight management strategies. www.naaso.org.

Ohayon MM. Prevalence and correlates of nonrestorative sleep complaints. *Arch Intern Med* 2005; 165(1):35–41.

Pick M. Insulin resistance in women. www.womentowomen.com/insulin resistance.

Problem sleepiness. National Institutes of Health National Heart, Lung, and Blood Institute 1997.

Rosedale R, Colman C. *The Rosedale Diet* (New York: Harper Resource, 2004).

Slumber weight away. *Prevention*, May 2005.

Spiegel K, Leproult R, L'Hermite-Balériaux M, Copinschi G, Penev P, Van Cauter E. Impact of sleep duration on the 24-hour leptin profile: relationships with sympatho-vagal balance, cortisol and TSH. *J Clin Endocrinol Metab* 2004; 89(11):5762–5771.

Spiegel K, Leproult R, Tasali E, Penev P, Van Cauter E. Sleep curtailment results in decreased leptin levels, elevated ghrelin levels and increased hunger and appetite. *Ann Intern Med* 2004; 141(11):846–850.

Spiegel K, Leproult R, Van Cauter E. Impact of sleep debt on metabolic and endocrine function. *Lancet* 1999; 354:1435–1439.

Stein R. Scientists finding out what losing sleep does to a body. *Washington Post,* Oct. 9, 2005.

Stuart N, Stuart R, Bjorbaek C, Guo L, Munzberg H. Leptin and obesity. *Proc Nat Acad Sci,* July 26, 2004.

Turner N. Total health and weight loss, the Truestar way. www.truestar health.com.

——— Sleep and weight loss. *Christian Post,* Feb. 22, 2006. www.christianpost. com/article/life/3216.

Van Cauter E et al. Age-related changes in slow wave sleep and REM sleep and relationship with growth hormone and cortisol levels in healthy men. *JAMA* 2000; 284:861–868, 880–881.

Van Cauter E et al. Impact of sleep length on the 24-hour leptin profile. Meeting of the Association of Professional Sleep Societies, Chicago, June 2001.

Van Cauter E, Latta F, Nedeltcheva A, Spiegel K, Leproult R, Vandenbril C, Weiss R, Mockel J, Legros J, Copinschi G. Reciprocal interactions between GH axis and sleep. *Growth Horm IGF Res* 2004; 14 Suppl A:S10–17.

Vorona R, Winn M, Babineau T, et al. Overweight and obese patients in a primary care population report less sleep than patients with a normal body mass index. *Arch Intern Med* 2005; 165:25–30.

Weight Loss Program. www.lindora.com/html/faqs.

Yildiz B, Suchard M, Wong M, McCann S, Licinio J. Alterations in the dynamics of circulating ghrelin, adiponectin, and leptin in human obesity. *Proc Natl Acad Sci* USA 2004; 101:10434–10439. PMID 15231.

CHAPTER TWO

The Burton Goldberg Group. *Alternative Medicine* (Puyallup, WA: Future Medicine Publishing, 1993).

Hornyak M, Voderholzer U, Hohagen F, Berger M, Riemann D. Magnesium therapy for periodic leg movements-related insomnia and restless legs syndrome: an open pilot study. *Sleep* 1998; 21(5):501–505.

Kahn A et al. Insomnia and cow's milk allergy in infants. *Pediatrics* 1985; 76(6): 880–884, in The Burton Goldberg Group, *Alternative Medicine* (Puyallup, WA: Future Medicine Publishing, 1993).

Mercola J, Droege R. Is insomnia wreaking havoc on your health? www.mercola.com, Feb. 7, 2004.

Murray M. *Encyclopedia of Nutritional Supplements* (Rocklin, CA: Prima Publishing, 1996).

Murray M, Pizzorno J. *Encyclopedia of Natural Medicine* 2nd ed. (Rocklin, CA: Prima Publishing, 1998).

Rosedale R. Insulin and its metabolic effects (July 14, 2001) and Leptin: how diabetes and obesity are linked (April 2, 2005), www.mercola.com.

30 Simple Tips to Help You Get to Sleep, www.well.com/user/mick/insomnia.

Whitaker J. *Health Healing* 2005; 15(11) and 15(12).

CHAPTER THREE

Adam D. *The Edge of Glory: Prayers in the Celtic Tradition* (Wilton, CT: Morehouse-Barlow, 1985), by permission of SPCK, London, England.

Breus M. Can't sleep? Insomnia types, causes, and treatments (Sept. 2004), www.webmd.com/content/Article/62/71841.htm.

Calbom C, Calbom J. *The Complete Cancer Cleanse* (Nashville, TN: Nelson, 2003).

———. *The Coconut Diet* (New York: Warner, 2005).

Calbom J. The choice response: changing your eating habits. Body, Mind and Spirit. *Choices* magazine.

———. Dealing with stress: a powerful immune builder. Body, Mind and Spirit. *Choices* magazine.

———. Positive actions bring positive results. Body, Mind and Spirit. *Choices* magazine.

———. Relax! you're already looking younger. Body, Mind and Spirit. *Choices* magazine.

———. Statistically speaking. Body, Mind and Spirit. *Choices* magazine.

———. Weak immune system? you may be "off purpose." Body, Mind and Spirit. *Choices* magazine.

Childre C, Martin H. *The Heartmath Solution.* (San Francisco, CA: Harper San Francisco, 1999).

Dwokson D, Sedona Training Associates. *The Sedona Method Course Workbook: Your Keys to Lasting Happiness, Abundance and Well Being* (Sedona, AR: Sedona Training Associates, 1991–2000).

HeartMath.org. www.heartmath.org.

Rauh S. Is your life running you ragged? (March 2005), www.webmd.com/content/Article/103/106976.htm.

Ricci A. Health professionals (2005), www.heartmath.com/health/professional/index.html.

Sewald P. *Wisdom from the Monastery: A Program of Spiritual Healing* (Old Saybrook, CT: Konecky and Konecky, 2003).

Web MD health. Sleep disorders: behavioral treatments (Sept. 2004), www.webmd.com.

———. Sleep disorders: insomnia (Sept. 2004), www.webmd.com.

———. Sleep: more important than you think (Oct. 2004), www.webmd.com.

Whittier, JG. The Brewing of Soma *The Atlantic Monthly,* April 1872.

CHAPTER FOUR

AARP. www.aarp.org.

American College of Sports Medicine, 50th Annual Meeting, San Francisco, CA. www.acsm.org/publications/newsreleases2003/exercisesleep060603.htm.

www.cyberparent.com/walks-walking/sleep-benefits.htm.

www.holisticonline.com.

Indiana University Health Center. The benefits of weight training. www.indiana.edu/~health/weightrn.

ipilates.com. www.i-pilates.com.

King A et al. Moderate-intensity exercise and self-rated quality of sleep in older adults. A randomized controlled trial. *JAMA* 1997; 277:32–37.

The Natural Health Perspective. http://naturalhealthperspective.com/exercise/pilates.

Pfitzinger P. The Pfitzinger Lab Report. www.pfitzinger.com/labreports/sleep (originally appeared in *Running Times* magazine).

Posen D. Stress management for patient and physician. *Can J Cont Med Ed,* April 1995.

Preston M. Cycling benefits and cautions. http://tms.ecol.net/fitness/bikepros.htm.

Rowbotham M. Exercise, not drugs, best insomnia Rx. *Medical Post,* Jan. 21, 1997.

Sansone L. *Walk Away the Pounds* (New York: Warner, 2005).

Singh N et al. A randomized controlled trial of the effect of exercise on sleep. *Sleep* 1997; 20:95–101.

Tworoger S et al. Effects of a yearlong moderate-intensity exercise and a stretching intervention on sleep quality in postmenopausal women. *Sleep* 2003; 26:830–836.

Walker M, Carter A. 33 ways the body responds to rebounding. www.healthbounce.com/33ways.

www.walking.about.com.

Weight Training Benefits and Cautions. http://tms.ecol.net/fitness/wghtpros.htm.

Youngerstedt S. Does exercise truly enhance sleep? *Physician Sportsmed* 1997; 25(10).

CHAPTER FIVE

Calbom C, Calbom J. *The Coconut Diet* (New York: Warner, 2005).

Elliott T. Lose fat while you sleep: turn your slumber into your best fat-burning session of the day with these seven nighttime supplements. *Muscle & Fitness,* June 2005.

Heinerman J. *Heinerman's Encyclopedia of Healing Juices* (Englewood Cliffs, NJ: Prentice Hall, 1994).

Lambert C. Deep into sleep. www.harvardmagazine.com/on-line/070587.

Lieberman S, Bruning M. *The Real Vitamin & Mineral Book* (New York: Avery, 1990).

Murray M. *Encyclopedia of Nutritional Supplements* (Rocklin, CA: Prima Publishing, 1996).

Murray M, Pizzorno J, Pizzorno L. *The Encyclopedia of Healing Foods* (New York: Atria Books: 2005).

Pitchford P. *Healing with Whole Foods* (Berkeley, CA: North Atlantic Books, 1993).

Rapp D. *Is This Your Child?* (New York: Quill, 1991).

Resetting the sleep clock. *Prevention's Healing with Vitamins.* www.mother-nature.com/Library/Bookshelf/Books.

Sleep problems could be elementary. Quarterly Report of Selected Research Projects, USDA Agricultural Research Service, April 1–June 30, 1988. In Murray F, Copper essential for healthy skin and hair. *Better Nutrition,* Feb. 1989.

CHAPTER SIX

Allen K, Frier B. Nocturnal hypoglycemia: clinical manifestations and therapeutic strategies toward prevention. *Endocr Pract* 2003; 9(6):530–543.

Barker J, Meletis C. The naturopathic approach to adrenal dysfunction. *Townsend Letter for Doctors and Patients,* Feb.–Mar. 2005.

Calbom C, Calbom J. *The Coconut Diet* (New York: Warner, 2005).

Kline M. Adrenal problems. Better Health Update 32, www.pacifichealthcenter.com/btr_health_updates.asp.

Mercola.com/September 22, 2005; *J Clin Endocrinol Metab* 2005; 90:4510–4515.

Murray M, Pizzorno J. *The Encyclopedia of Natural Medicine* (Rocklin, CA: Prima Publishing, 1998).

Sleephealthyresources.com. www.newtechpub.com.

Sohmiya M, Kato Y. Fluctuations of physical function affected by sleep-awake rhythm–endocrine system. *Nippon Rinsho* (Japanese) 1998; 56(2):342–347.

Tamas L, Xiao-Bing G. Input organization and plasticity of hypocretin neurons: possible clues to obesity's association with insomnia. *Cell Metab* 2005; 1(4): 279–286.

Vgontzas A et al. Chronic insomnia is associated with nyctohemeral activation of the hypothalamic-pituitary-adrenal axis: clinical implications. *J Clin Endocrinol Metab* 2001; 86:3787–3794.

Wilson J. *Adrenal Fatigue* (Petaluma, CA: Smart Publications, 2001).

CHAPTER SEVEN

Allen K, Frier B. Nocturnal hypoglycemia: clinical manifestations and therapeutic strategies toward prevention. *Endocrinol Pract* 2003; 9(6):530–543.

Beers T. Flexible schedules and shift work: replacing the "9-to-5" workday? *Mon Labor Rev* 2000; 123:33–40.

Bolton S. *J Orthomol Psych* 13(1).

Diagnostic and Statistical Manual of Mental Disorders, 4th ed. (Washington, DC: American Psychiatric Association, 2000).

Kantrowitz B. The Quest for Rest. *Newsweek,* Apr. 24, 2006.

Lutz E. Restless legs, anxiety, and caffeinism. Clin Psych Sept. 1978; 693–698.

MayoClinic.com. Tips for shift workers. www.mayoclinic.com/health/shift-work.

Mercola.com. Lack of Daylight May Cause Insomnia. July 7, 2001.

Mishima K et al. Diminished melatonin secretion in the elderly caused by insufficient environmental illumination. *J Clin Endocrinol Metab* 2001; 86:129–134.

National Sleep Foundation. 2002 Sleep in America Poll. Washington, DC: National Sleep Foundation, 2002. www.nhlbi.nih.gov/health/public/sleep/rls.txt. Accessed April 25, 2005.

Problem sleepiness. National Institutes of Health National Heart, Lung, and Blood Institute. 1997.

Psychology Today online, Nov. 13, 2003 (3116).

Restless Legs Syndrome Foundation. www.rls.org.

Shaw G. To sleep, perchance to sleep soundly. www.aolsvc.health.webmd.aol.com.

Sleephealthyresources.com. www.healthyresources.com.

Sleeping pills: fact and fiction. Quest 2000; 7(5). www.mdausa.org/publications/Quest/q75sleepingpills.html.

Sleeping pills: a prescription for better sleep? www.mayoclinic.com/health/sleeping-pills.

Understanding insomnia medications. www.emedicinehealth.com.

CHAPTER EIGHT

The menu plan was adapted from Calbom C, Calbom J. *The Coconut Diet* (New York: Warner, 2005).

www.shakeoffthesugar.net/article1042.

INDEX

acupuncture, 144, 145
acute insomnia, 140
acyanthopanax obovatus root, 110
Adam, David, 60–61
adenosine triphosphate (ATP), ix, 94, 115
adrenal cortical cell extracts, 133, 204
adrenal dysfunction, 123–34, 146
  correcting, 127, 129–33
  stressors triggering, 125
  symptoms, 126
Adrenal Fatigue (Wilson), 127, 132, 133
adrenal function tests, 128
adrenal glands, 120–34, 146
adrenaline, 16, 121, 154
adrenal support supplements, 133, 142,
  204
adrenocorticotropin, 121
aerobic exercises, 83–93
agave syrup, 183
age (aging)
  growth hormone and, 25
  insomnia and, 147
alarm clocks, 39, 41
alcohol, 30, 114
  adrenal dysfunction and, 130
  restless legs syndrome and, 159–60
  sleep apnea and, 158
allergies, 40, 117, 158–59
almonds, 31, 101–2, 136, 156, 170
aluminum, 33, 115
Ambien, 150–51
amino acids, 103–4
AMSH, 12
anger, Sedona Method for, 68
animal proteins
  to avoid, 183–84
  CLA levels and, 105–6
  to eat, 167–68, 174–76

antacids, 115
antidepressants, 82, 159–60
antihistamines, 150–51
anxiety, 50–52, 138–39. *See also* stress
  management
  understanding source, and letting go,
  67–71
apathy, Sedona Method for, 68
appetite-stimulating hormones, 3, 9–11,
  27. *See also* ghrelin
appetite-suppressing hormones, 3, 9–11,
  27. *See also* leptin
appreciation from the heart, 72–74
Armour, J. Andrew, 71
ashwagandha, 110
ATP (adenosine triphosphate), ix, 94, 115
audio sleep programs, 143
Ayas, Najib T., 2

back, sleeping on your, 38
basic meditation, 57
baths, before bedtime, 37
B-complex vitamins, 108–10, 132, 136, 142
beans (legumes), 167, 171–74, 179
bedding, 41, 42
bedroom environment, 36, 37, 39, 41, 42
bedroom temperature, 33
bedtime routine, 29, 162
  avoiding drugs late night, 40
  light snack before, 31
  regular and consistent schedule, 29, 158,
  162
  relaxing and winding down, 37
  sniffing lavender, 34
beef
  to avoid, 183
  CLA levels and, 105–6
  to eat, 167, 174–75

behaviors, reframing, 63–65
Benedict, Saint, 62
Benson, Herbert, 58
benzodiazepines, 150–51
berries, 178
best food choices, 100–103, 174–83
beverages
    to avoid, 114–19, 184
    to drink, 168, 176–77
bicycling, 92
bioflavonoids, 131–32, 142
birch sugar, 171, 181, 203
blood pressure, and adrenal function tests,
    128
blood sugar (glucose), 17–18, 127, 129, 152–
    56. *See also* nocturnal hypoglycemia
    cortisol and, 23, 127
    foods to avoid for, 118–19, 156
    foods to eat for, 141–42, 156
    glycemic index and, 182
    managing, 153–56
body alignment, 41–42, 147
body temperature, 33
Bolton, Sanford, 129
bone density, and growth hormone, 24–25
brain entrainment, 56–58
breads, 190
breathing exercises, 34, 53, 95–98, 142
butter, 169, 178

caffeine, 29–30, 115, 116
    adrenal dysfunction and, 124, 129–30
calcium, 32–33, 105, 108, 142
California poppy, 111
calming agents, 110–13
Calms Forté, 142
carbohydrates. *See* complex carbohydrates;
    refined carbohydrates
catnip, 111
celery, 100
Celtic prayers, 60–61
chamomile (tea), 32, 111
chanting, 56–58
chattering mind, 51
cheeses, 168
chi (energy), 143–45, 184
chia seeds, 100

chicken, 101–2, 168
Chinese medicine
    foods aiding sleep, 100–101
    insomnia in, 143–45
chiropractic care, 147
choice responses, 74–77
cholesterol, and aerobic exercise, 91
chromium, 106
chronic sleep deprivation (insomnia), 8–9,
    140
cigarettes, 29–30, 116
    restless legs syndrome and, 159–60
    sleep apnea and, 157–58
circadian rhythms, 25, 81, 82
CLA (conjugated linoleic acid), 105–6,
    174–75
cleansing, 146–47
    1-Day Vegetable Juice Cleanse, 188–89
    products, resources, 203–4
closing the day with prayer, 59–61
Coconut Diet, The (Calbom), 103, 148, 165
coconut oil, 103, 135, 169, 177, 203
cod-liver oil, 21, 136
coenzyme A (CoA), 131
Coffea Cruda, 112
coffee. *See* caffeine
cognitive behavioral therapy, 149
colon cleanse, resources, 203
colors, bedroom, 42
complex carbohydrates, 102–3
conjugated linoleic acid (CLA), 105–6,
    174–75
copper, 106–7
cortisol, 22–24, 125, 127
    adrenal dysfunction and, 146
    defined, 10
    stress and immunity, 46
    weight gain and, 124
cotton bedding, 41
counting sheep, 38
cravings, 14, 15–16, 155, 165
cycling, 92
Czeisler, Charles, 9

dairy products, 168
dairy substitutes, 184
dance aerobics, 93

dark rooms, 36, 161–62
deep-breathing exercises, 34, 53, 96–97, 142
detox, 33, 146–47. *See also* cleansing
diabetes, 19
Diabetes Prevention Program (DPP), 19
diet, 99–119. *See also* menu plan
    adrenal dysfunction and, 127–28
    foods aiding sleep, 100–103, 174–81
    foods to avoid, 114–19, 183–87
    glycemic index and, 182
    growth hormone and, 25
    leptin and insulin resistance and, 20–21
    sleeping tips, 30–32, 40
digestion, 31–32, 34, 147
Doghramji, Karl, 151
dream-disturbed sleep (nightmares),
    144–45
drinks. *See* alcohol; beverages
drugs, 116–17. *See also* supplements
    restless leg syndrome and, 159–60
    sleeping pills, 149–51
    taking before bedtime, 40

earplugs, 39, 161–62
eating. *See* diet; menu plan
*Edge of Glory, The: Prayers in the Celtic
    Tradition* (Adam), 60–61
eggs, 167, 169, 175
electromagnetic fields (EMFs), 39–40
emotional indigestion, 31–32
emotions, and sleep, 50, 52
endocrine system, 120–36
epigallocatechin gallate (EGCG), 176
epinephrine, 131
estrogen, xii, 162, 163
exercise, 42–43, 79–98
    aerobic, 83–93
    best time for, 81
    cortisol and, 130
    growth hormone and, 25
    leptin and insulin resistance and, 20
    for persons with physical limitations,
      88–89
    stretching and breathing, 94–98
    weight and resistance training, 93–95
exercise equipment, in the bedroom, 42
expressing feelings, 70–71

Fast-Track 1-Day Vegetable Juice Cleanse,
    188–89
fast walking, 90–91
fats (oils)
    adrenal dysfunction and, 127, 129
    to avoid, 184
    best, 169, 177–78
    ghrelin and, 22
    growth hormone and, 24–25
    insulin resistance and, 17, 21
    leptin resistance and, 15–16, 21
    thyroid function and, 135
fear, Sedona Method for, 68
feng shui, 41–42
fight-or-flight response, 23
fish, 21, 107, 175–76
flax seeds, 21
fluid intake, 40, 176–77, 190
food. *See* diet; menu plan
food allergies and intolerances, 40, 117,
    158–59
food colorings and dyes, 117
food cravings, 14, 15–16, 155, 165
food products, resources, 203
forgiveness, 61–62
fruits, 21, 169, 178–79, 185
full-spectrum light, 82, 161

GABA (gamma-aminobutyric acid), 103–4
gallbladder cleanse, resources, 203
GH (growth hormone), 10, 24–25, 90
ghee, 178
ghrelin, 10, 15, 21–22
glasses, rose-colored, 36–37
glucagon, 175
glucose. *See* blood sugar
glutamine, 103–4
glycemic index, 182
glycemic load, 182
glycine, 103–4
God (Higher Power), 58
goitrogens, 136
good night's sleep
    defined, 5–6
    practical tips for, 28–43
grains, 103, 167, 168–69, 185
grass-fed beef, 105–6, 165, 167, 174–75

green tea, 176
Gregorian chants, 56–58
grief, Sedona Method for, 68
growth hormone (GH), 10, 24–25, 90
Gui Pi Tang, 144

Haas, Elson M., 107, 129–30
health centers, 205–7
heart (heart intelligence), 71–74
heavy meals, late in day, 30–31, 163
heavy metal detox program, 33
herbal sedatives, 110–12
Holmes, Thomas H., 48–49
hops, 111
hormone replacement therapy, 163
hormones, xii, 2–3, 148. *See also specific hormones*
    adrenal function tests, 128
    links among sleep, weight loss, and, 9–11
hydrochloric acid, 131, 147
5-hydroxytryptophan (5-HTP), 110, 113, 176
hyperglycemia (high blood sugar), 119
hypertension, and aerobic exercise, 91
hypnotics, 150–51
hypocretin, 134
hypoglycemia (low blood sugar). *See* nocturnal hypoglycemia
hypopnea (shallow breathing), 156–59
hypothalamus, 10, 12, 22, 120–22, 134
hypothalamus extract, 134
hypothyroidism, 135–36, 148

ignatia, 112
immunity, and stress, 45–50
indigestion, 31–32, 147
inositol, 110
insomnia, 137–51
    adrenal dysfunction and, 123–24, 146
    anxiety and, 51
    cortisol and, 23–24
    defined, 139
    exercise and, 82
    getting at roots of, 145–48
    helpful remedies for, 141–43
    menopause and sweets, 118
    resources, 207
    sleeping pills for, 149–51
    stress and, 48
    in traditional Chinese medicine, 143–45
    types of, 140, 143
insulin, 10, 17–18, 23, 121
insulin-like growth factor 1 (IGF-1), 24
insulin resistance, 17–21
interferon, 46
intermittent insomnia, 140
iodine (salt), 130–31, 136, 180
iron, 107, 148
Is My Child Overtired? (Wilkoff), 4

jet lag, 42
jobs, shift work sleep disorder (SWSD), 161–62
jogging, 90–91
journals, 39
juicers, resources, 203
juicing, 187–89
jujaba leaf, 112
jujube seeds, 100
juncus effuses leaf, 111

Kawai, Kirio, 15
King, Lou Ann, 59

Lancet, 18, 23
large meals, late in day, 30–31, 163
lavender, 34, 142
legumes, 167, 171–74, 179
leptin, 11–17
    defined, 10
    nocturnal hypoglycemia and, 154
    normal levels, 13
    role of, 13
leptin resistance, 13–17
    reversing, 19–21
    symptoms, 13, 16
letting go of stress, 67–71
lettuce (juice), 32, 101, 172
Levenson, Lester, 67–71
licorice, 132
Life Balance Quiz, 46–47
lifestyle choice responses, 74–77

light, 42, 82, 160–61
  endocrine system, sleep, and, 122
lighting, in the bedroom, 37
liquor, 30, 114
  adrenal dysfunction and, 130
  restless legs syndrome and, 159–60
  sleep apnea and, 158
liver cleansing, 146–47, 155, 203
"living from your heart," 72–74
Lo Han Guo, 171, 181
Lord's Prayer, 59
low blood sugar. *See* nocturnal hypoglycemia
low-carb diet, 166
low thyroid function, 135–36, 148
Lunesta, 150–51
lust, Sedona Method for, 68
Luvox, 151
lymphasizers, 88–89, 203
lymph system, rebounding for, 86–87

McTiernan, Anne, 162
magnesium, 32–33, 107–8, 131–32, 142
manganese, 134
marijuana, 117
massages, 36
mattresses, 41
medications, 116–17. *See also* supplements
  restless leg syndrome and, 159–60
  sleeping pills, 149–51
  taking before bedtime, 40
meditation, 57
melatonin, 112–13, 121
  rose-colored glasses and, 36–37
  sunlight, sleep, and, 122, 160
menopausal sleep problems, 118, 162–63
Menopause Without Medicine (Ojeda),
  118
mental health, and stress, 45–46, 48, 50
mental indigestion, 31–32
menu plan, 164–96
  basic guidelines, 190
  best food choices, 174–83
  dinners helping you sleep, 196
  foods to avoid, 183–87
  foods to eat, 166–74
  juicing, 187–89

  sample menus, 191–95
  servings guidelines, 167
Mercola, Joseph, 29
metabolism, 3–4
Mignot, Emmanuel, 1–2
milk products, 168
milk substitutes, 184
mitochondria, 93–94
morning exercise, 81
movement, 79–80. *See also* exercise
MSG (monosodium glutamate), 118, 130
mulberries, 101
muscle development
  growth hormone and, 24–25
  weight training for, 93–94
muscle relaxation technique, 55–56
mushrooms, 172–73
music, 37–38, 39, 56–58

Naiman, Rubin, 123
naps (napping), 9, 29, 162
nasal problems, 148, 158–59
natural sedatives, 110–13
negative thoughts, 54, 67–71
New Detox Diet, The (Haas), 129–30
niacinamide (vitamin B_3), 109
nicotine. *See* smoking
nightmares, 144–45
nocturnal hypoglycemia, 152–56
  alcohol and, 114
  chromium supplements for, 106
  correcting, 156
  light snacks before bedtime for, 31
  managing blood sugar, 153–56
  symptoms, 152, 153
non-rapid-eye-movement sleep (NREM),
  6–7
nonrestorative sleep (NRS), 6
norepinephrine, 131
nutritional supplements. *See* supplements
nuts (nut butters), 21, 101–2, 107, 136,
  167, 170–71
nux vomica, 113

oats, 103
obstructive sleep apnea (OSA), 156–59
oils. *See* fats

Ojeda, Linda, 118
olive oil, 135, 169, 177
omega-3 fatty acids, 21, 175–76
1-Day Vegetable Juice Cleanse, 188–89
orexin, 134
organic cotton bedding, 41
organic produce, 179–80
OSA (obstructive sleep apnea), 156–59
overactive mind, 51
oysters, 101, 107

pancreas, 17, 18, 121
pantothenic acid (vitamin B₅), 109, 132
passionflower, 111
Paxil, 82, 159–60
peanuts, 136
pearlicium, 111
Penland, James C., 106, 115
personal relaxation formula, 77
pesticides, 179–80
physical limitations and disabilities,
     exercise for persons with, 88–89
Pilates, 94–95
pillows, 41
pineal gland, 120–22
pituitary gland, 22, 24, 120–22
PMS symptoms, menu plan for, 165
polyunsaturated fats, 135, 184
pork, 183
positional tension, 35
positive attitude, 54–58
positive behaviors, 63–65
potatoes, 178–79, 187
prayer, 59–61
pride, Sedona Method for, 68–69
primary insomnia, 140
progressive muscle relaxation, 55–56
Prozac, 82
psychological side of stress management,
     54–58
psychological stressors, 48–49, 50, 54, 125
psychophysiological insomnia, 51, 138–39,
     140
purpose in life, 66–67
pyridoxine (vitamin B₆), 109

Quiz, Life Balance, 46–47

Rahe, Richard H., 48–49
rapid-eye-movement (REM) sleep, 5, 6–7,
     150
reading in bed, 37
rebounding, 86–88
refined carbohydrates, 30, 31, 118–19
     adrenal dysfunction and, 127, 129
     insulin resistance and, 17–18
     nocturnal hypoglycemia and, 156
reframing, 63–65
relaxation, 45, 55–58. *See also* stress
     management
     breathing exercises, 34, 53, 95–98, 142
     massages, 36
     personal formula for, 77
     soothing music, 37–38, 39, 56–58
     techniques for, 55–58
     visualizations, 35–36
     winding down before sleep, 37
religious practices, 58–63
REM (rapid-eye-movement) sleep, 5, 6–7,
     150
Rescue Remedy, 113, 143
resistance training, 93–95
resources, 202–7
restless leg syndrome (RLS), 159–60
restorative sleep, 5–6
rose-colored glasses, 36–37
Rosedale, Ron, 15, 153–54, 155
Roth, Thomas, 149
routine for bedtime, 29, 162
     avoiding drugs late night, 40
     light snack before, 31
     regular and consistent schedule, 29, 158,
         162
     relaxing and winding down, 37
     sniffing lavender, 34
Rozerem, 150–51
running, 90–91

saliva hormone tests, 128
salt (iodine), 130–31, 136, 180
Sansone, Leslie, 85
saunas, before bedtime, 37
schedule, sleep, 29, 158, 162
secondary insomnia, 140
Sedona Method, 67–71

seeds (seed butters), 167, 170–71
serotonin, 31, 141–42
shallow breathing (hypopnea), 156–59
shift work sleep disorder (SWSD), 161–62
showers, before bedtime, 37
Simon, David, 29
Sinupret, 148
sinus problems, 148, 158–59
sleep
  amount needed, 8, 28
  emotions and, 50, 52
  links among hormones, weight loss, and, 9–11
  practical tips for, 28–43
  stages of, 6–7
  sunlight, endocrine system, and, 122
  value of refreshing, 5–6
sleep aids, 110–13, 205
sleep anxiety. *See* anxiety
sleep apnea, 156–59
Sleep Away the Pounds Menu Plan. *See* menu plan
sleep deprivation (deficit), 27–28
  cortisol and, 23
  endocrine system and, 121
  insulin sensitivity and, 17, 18–19
  making up, 8–9
sleep disorders, 137–63. *See also* insomnia
  lack of sunlight exposure, 160–61
  menopausal sleep problems, 118, 162–63
  nocturnal hypoglycemia, 152–56
  restless leg syndrome, 159–60
  shift work sleep disorder, 161–62
  sleep apnea and snoring, 156–59
sleep habits, 4–5, 28
sleep hygiene, practical tips, 28–43
sleeping pills, 149–51
sleeplessness. *See* insomnia
sleep memories, 35
sleep research (studies), 1–2, 4–5, 10, 27
sleep tapes, 143
sleeptime routine. *See* bedtime routine
slow-wave sleep (SWS), 7
smoking, 29–30, 116
  restless legs syndrome and, 159–60
  sleep apnea and, 157–58
snacks (snacking), 31, 155, 186

snoring, 39, 156–59
soy (soybeans), 136
spices, 180
spinal structure imbalances, 147
spiritual side of stress management, 58–63
SSRIs (selective serotonin reuptake inhibitors), 82, 159–60
stage 1 sleep, 7, 23–24, 158
stage 2 sleep (theta sleep), 7
stage 3 and 4 sleep (delta sleep), 7
stage 5 sleep (REM sleep), 5, 6–7
stages of sleep, 6–7
staring at one spot, 35
step aerobics, 93
stevia, 171, 181
Stickgold, Robert, 4
stimulating activities, close to bedtime, 38
stress
  adrenal dysfunction and, 123–24, 127
  digestion and, 147
  immunity and, 45–50
  understanding source, and letting go, 67–71
stressful events, 48–49, 50
stress management, 45, 50–62
  personal relaxation formula, 77
  physical side of, 52–53
  psychological side of, 54–58
  Sedona Method for, 67–71
  spiritual side of, 58–63
stress signals, 54
stretching, 94–98
sugars, 30, 31, 118–19, 127, 129, 156, 187
sugar substitutes (sweeteners), 21, 167, 171, 180–81, 183, 187
sunlight, 42, 82, 160–61
  endocrine system, sleep, and, 122
supplements, 32–33, 103–10
  correcting adrenal function, 131–33
  resources, 204
  for thyroid health, 136
suppressing feelings, 70–71
sweeteners (sugar substitutes), 21, 167, 171, 180–81, 183, 187
sweets, 14, 15–16, 118–19, 155, 186
swimming, 89, 92–93
SWSD (shift work sleep disorder), 161–62

Tasali, Esra, 17
temperature, of bedroom, 33
Teng Yin, 145
tension, 35
testosterone, xii, 25
Theophan, Saint, 59–60
thiamin (vitamin B₁), 109
thumb, clasping left, 35
thyroid medications, 116–17, 204
thyroid problems, 135–36, 148
Tian Ma Gou, 145
Tian Wang Bu Xin Dan, 145
tobacco. *See* smoking
to-do lists, before going to bed, 39
toe wiggling, 33–34
Tomatis, Alfred, 56–58
tossing and turning, in bed, 145
traditional Chinese medicine (TCM)
    foods aiding sleep, 100–101
    insomnia in, 143–45
Trinder, John, 91
tryptophan-rich foods, 31, 101–2, 141–42,
    156
tummy rubbing, 34
turkey, 31, 101–2, 141–42, 156
21-Day Sleep Away the Pounds Menu
    Plan. *See* menu plan
tyramine-containing foods, 119
tyrosine, 102–3, 176

vagus nerve, 27
valerian root, 111
Valium, 150
Van Cauter, Eve, 2, 14, 18–19, 21
Vegetable Juice Cleanse, Fast-Track 1-Day,
    188–89
vegetable juices (juicing), 176, 187–89
vegetables, 33, 101, 102–3
    to avoid, 187
    to eat, 101, 102–3, 171–74, 178–79
    leptin resistance and, 21
    servings guidelines, 167
    thyroid problems and, 136
visualizations, 35–36

vitamins, 32–33, 103–10
    correcting adrenal function, 131–33
    resources, 204
    for thyroid health, 136
vitamin A, 136
vitamin B₁, 109
vitamin B₃, 109
vitamin B₅, 109, 132
vitamin B₆, 109
vitamin C, 107, 131–32, 142
vitamin D, 82

Wadden, Thomas, 4–5
wakefulness, and cortisol, 23–24
Walk Away the Pounds (Sansone), 85
walking, 84–85
    fast, 90–91
warm feet, 33
water aerobics, 89, 92–93
water, drinking, 40, 176–77, 190
weight loss, 40
    leptin and insulin resistance and, 20
    links among sleep, hormones, and,
        9–11
    sleep apnea and, 157
weight training, 93–95
Wen Dan Tang, 144
Werbach, Melvyn R., 32
white chestnut, 113, 143
whole grains, 103, 165, 169, 185
wiggling the toes, 33–34
Wilkoff, Will, 4
Wilson, James L., 127, 132, 133
Winkelman, John, 9
winter, sleeping tips, 29
work sleep disorder, shift, 161–62

Xanax, 150
xylitol (birch sugar), 171, 181, 203

Youngstedt, Shawn D., 82

Ziziphas jujaba leaf, 112
Zoloft, 82